TEACHING TOMORROW'S NURSES

A TECHNOLOGY-ENHANCED APPROACH

National League for Nursing

TEACHING TOMORROW'S NURSES

A TECHNOLOGY-ENHANCED APPROACH

Edited by:

Jennifer O'Rourke, PhD, APRN, CHSE

Andrew Bobal, EdD

. Wolters Kluwer

Philadelphia · Baltimore · New York · London
Buenos Aires · Hong Kong · Sydney · Tokyo

Vice President and Segment Leader, Health Learning, and Practice: Julie K. Stegman
Director, Nursing Education and Practice Content: Jamie Blum
Senior Development Editor: Meredith L. Brittain
Marketing Manager: Greta Swanson
Editorial Assistant: Sara Thul
Manager, Graphic Arts and Design: Steve Druding
Art Director: Jennifer Clements
Production Project Manager: Bridgett Dougherty
Manufacturing Coordinator: Margie Orzech
Prepress Vendor: Aptara, Inc.

O'Rourke, J., & Bobal, A. (2025). *Teaching tomorrow's nurses: A technology-enhanced approach.* National League for Nursing.

9 8 7 6 5 4 3 2 1

Printed in the United States of America

Library of Congress Cataloging-in-Publication Data

978-1-9752-4827-7

Cataloging-in-Publication data available on request from publisher.

MPP0624

To my parents, Lawrence and Patricia O'Rourke, both writers and editors by trade and passion, for their constant support and enthusiasm for each and every project I have taken on.

To my children, Nora, Jamie, and Bailey, for providing me joy, drive, and balance. Love you to the moon and back.

—Jennifer O'Rourke

To my parents, Jim and Jessica Bobal, for always pushing me to do my best and supporting me in everything I have done and continue to pursue.

To my amazing wife, Sarah, for continuing to support all the craziness of our wonderful life. To my children, Max and Emry, who remind me to continue to be the best person I can be and not to take things too seriously.

Finally, to my extended family, which consists of retired and current educators, current and retired nurses, and multiple other extremely valuable professions, thank you for pushing me and setting the stage to be great. I love you all more than you will ever know!

—Andrew Bobal

About the Editors

Jennifer O'Rourke, PhD, APRN, CHSE is an associate professor and the associate dean of the Parkinson School of Health Sciences and Public Health at Loyola University Chicago. She graduated with her undergraduate degree in nursing from Villanova University and received her master's and doctorate from the University of Illinois–Chicago. She is on the editorial board for the National League for Nursing (NLN) *Education Perspectives* journal and was a member of the 2016 NLN Simulation Lead program. She has published and presented widely in the field of nursing education, with over 50 articles in peer-reviewed journals. She is an author on the *National Organization of Nurse Practitioner Faculties (NONPF) 2023 Guide to Developing Simulations: A Step-By-Step Approach* and served as a peer reviewer of the NONPF *Simulation Guidelines & Best Practices: For Nurse Practitioner Education*. She also coedited the 2022 NONPF podcast series, *Simulation Podcast Series in the Trenches: Confessions and Pearls of NP Simulationists*. Most recently, she served as coeditor of the reimagined NLN SIRC foundations and deeper dive simulation courses. She has served as a consultant for the NLN since 2019.

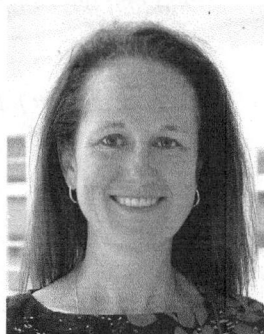

Andrew Bobal, EdD is an educator with over 14 years of experience in K-12 and higher education. With a background as a STEM classroom teacher and technology leader, he is currently an instructional designer and adjunct professor at Widener University School of Nursing in Chester, Pennsylvania. After graduating with a degree in Elementary Education from Bloomsburg University of Pennsylvania, Andrew started his career in 2009 in Clarksville, Tennessee, as a fourth-grade STEM teacher at Minglewood Elementary. There he was recognized for his outstanding teaching, receiving multiple accolades. The classroom sparked his interest in technology integration in education. In 2013 he received his master's degree in instructional technology from Austin Peay State University in Clarksville. After completing his master's degree, he sought a position that focused on technology integration and working with others to better their instructional pedagogy. His work at Widener University in the School of Nursing started in 2015 and added to his drive to be a leader within the field. In May 2020 he graduated from Widener with an EdD in K-12 educational leadership. His successful work at Widener led him to a professional relationship with the National League for Nursing (NLN), where he currently serves as the instructional technologist/designer in the NLN's Center for Innovation in Education Excellence. He has presented at multiple conferences, both national and international, and he has authored numerous publications.

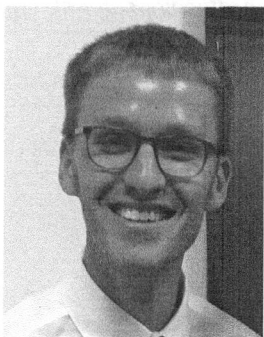

About the Contributors

Matthew Byrne, PhD, RN, CNE works on clinical technology projects across the Mayo Clinic enterprise. He is helping shape next-generation clinical technologies that will realize the true value nurses bring to health care while also maximizing how technology can best support practice. He has taught undergraduate and graduate nursing for almost 20 years in the clinical, simulation laboratory, classroom, and online environments. He is passionate about teaching and advancing educational technology through best practices and working to best meet students where they are not only cognitively but also in terms of their personal identity and preferences. He has published his own e-learning design model focused on promoting high-quality and high-impact significant e-learning experiences. He teaches on a variety of education and informatics topics with an emphasis on educational and clinical decision support. He serves as the emerging technologies editor for *Nursing Education Perspectives* and reviews for multiple journals.

Emily Chin, PhD, MSN, RNC-MNN, C-EFM is an Assistant Professor and Program Director of the four-year BSN program, who joined the Marcella Niehoff School of Nursing (MNSON) faculty in 2012. She has taught courses across all levels of the BSN program and has previously served as advisor to the Student Nurse Association of Illinois at Loyola and the Nursing Student Council. She serves on two HRSA-funded projects promoting inclusive excellence at the MNSON. Within the CARE (Collaboration, Access, Resources, and Equity) Pathway to the BSN, she oversees the first-year seminars, helping students transition to the nursing program. Within the Social Determinants of Health—Nursing Providing Access to Healthcare project, she works closely with a local high school to enhance students' understanding of nursing and expand recruitment into the profession. Additionally, she maintains clinical practice as an obstetrical staff nurse.

Matthew Chrisman, PhD is an Associate Professor at the University of Missouri–Kansas City School of Nursing and Health Studies. He has been the principal investigator or coinvestigator on numerous funded studies examining topics related to health promotion in education. He has mentored numerous graduate and undergraduate students, which has resulted in several nursing education-focused publications, including a review of escape rooms, examination of nursing faculty perceptions of prelicensure education, and incivility in nursing.

Rebecca G. Davis, EdD, RN, CNE, CNE-cl is a Clinical Associate Professor at the University of Alabama in Huntsville College of Nursing. She has been teaching since 2007 in the clinical, classroom, simulation, and online learning environments. She teaches medical-surgical nursing in the prelicensure BSN program, nursing education courses at the MSN level, and chairs/serves on PhD dissertation committees. She serves as the curriculum chair for UAH College of Nursing's four undergraduate programs. Her research interests include nurse's development of clinical judgment, innovative teaching-learning strategies, nursing curriculum transformation, and transfer of learning into clinical practice. She earned her BSN from the University of Alabama in Huntsville in 1998, and her MSN in Nursing as an adult health clinical nurse specialist in 2008, also from the University of Alabama in Huntsville. She earned her EdD in instructional leadership in August 2020 from the University of Alabama. She is certified as both an academic nurse educator and an academic clinical nurse educator.

Laura Gonzalez, PhD, MSN, RNC-MNN, C-EFM is an Assistant Professor and Director of Part-Time Undergraduate Faculty who joined the Marcella Niehoff School of Nursing Faculty at Loyola University Chicago in 2012. She has taught clinicals and courses across the BSN program. She has lectured both in person and virtual in the classroom. As Director of Undergraduate Faculty, she oversees part-time faculty to ensure they are prepared to enhance the student's education. She also serves at the Institute for Transformative Interprofessional Education to promote interprofessional collaboration. She continues to maintain clinical practice as a clinical quality improvement specialist. Her research focus is on maternal health and perinatal mental health.

Elaine D. Kauschinger, PhD, APRN, FAANP is an Assistant Professor of Clinical Nursing at the Duke University School of Nursing, serving as the primary care adolescent and adult course coordinator. She is a board-certified family nurse practitioner with a diverse clinical background in family practice, substance abuse, occupational health, and infectious diseases. Her area of scholarship is in virtual patient and artificial intelligence–assisted simulation. She has authored several book chapters on virtual patient simulation, primary care, nursing education, and board review preparation for nurse practitioners. Her expertise in virtual patient simulation technology has led to her appointment as an invited member of the Simulation Committee for the National Organization of Nurse Practitioner Faculties, where she has also served as the chair of the Simulation Special Interest Group. She is also a Fellow of the American Association of Nurse Practitioners.

Kevin Mazor, PhD is an Assistant Professor who joined the Loyola University Chicago Marcella Niehoff School of Nursing (MNSON) faculty in 2017. He has bachelor's degrees in biochemistry and nutrition from Michigan State University, and a PhD in molecular nutrition from Cornell University. As a graduate researcher he investigated the unique role that methionine has on the regulation of protein synthesis. As a member of the MNSON, he has taught microbiology, nutrition, and physiology to first- and second-year students in the BSN program, while also serving as an advisor to the Student Nurse Association of Illinois at Loyola. He serves as an advisor to undergraduate nursing researchers who have completed research projects on a variety of topics, including hand hygiene practices during the pandemic and the impact the pandemic had on the lifestyles of diabetic students. He consistently works to integrate new technologies and practices into his compassionate pedagogical approaches with the aim of maximizing student learning while minimizing unproductive stress.

Michelle C. Moulton, DNP, RN, CHSE, CNE is the Director of the Center for Clinical Excellence at the University of Maryland St. Joseph Medical Center in Towson,

Maryland. Michelle celebrates over 22 years in nursing and 14 years of academic teaching experience at the state and national level. Dr. Moulton recently returned to the acute care practice setting to lead initiatives and build programs through teaming that advance nursing practice in the service of patient care excellence. Michelle's specialty areas in nursing education and practice include professional development, neuroscience informed teaching, experiential teaching-learning strategies, and debriefing. Her doctoral work focused on implementing simulation-based education to improve nurses' response to patient deterioration using situational awareness skills.

Rachel Onello, PhD, RN, CHSE, CNE, CNE-cl, CNL, ANEF is recognized nationally as an expert in evidence-based teaching practices grounded in the cognitive science of learning. Her work in shaping the development, facilitation, and evaluation of national faculty development initiatives has contributed to advancing the art and science of good teaching across learning environments. With a focus on educational design, she seeks to build nurse educators' skills in implementing best practices of teaching and learning that transforms student thinking and promotes excellence in teaching. She has taught in baccalaureate, entry-level master's, and graduate programs since 2008, focusing on designing, implementing, and evaluating didactic, clinical, and simulation-based education. She teaches across online, classroom, and clinical learning environments, integrating evidence-based neuroscience principles in teaching and learning pedagogy with a focus on psychological safety. She received training in psychological safety, simulation, and debriefing through Harvard's Center for Medical Simulation and the Peter M. Winter Institute for Simulation, Education, and Research. She is an NLN Jonas Scholar emeritus and a fellow in the National League for Nursing Academy of Nursing Education. She holds national certifications as a Certified Healthcare Simulation Educator, Certified Nurse Educator, Certified Clinical Nurse Educator, and Certified Clinical Nurse Leader.

Sarah E. Patel, PhD, RN, C-EFM is an Assistant Professor at the University of Missouri–Kansas City School of Nursing and Health Studies. She enjoys teaching undergraduate and graduate nursing students. She received her Doctor of Philosophy in Nursing degree at the University of Missouri–Kansas City. Her dissertation research focused on the relationship of staff nurse incivility and undergraduate nursing students' sense of belonging in the nursing profession. She has served as author and coauthor on several articles focused on nursing education and integrating innovation teaching modalities, including escape rooms and telehealth modalities. Her areas of research include chronic pelvic pain in women, innovative teaching strategies in nursing education, incivility in nursing, and sense of belonging in nursing.

Emily A. Reinkemeyer, MSN, RN, CPAN received her BSN from Missouri State University and her MSN in Nursing Education from University of Missouri–Kansas City, where she published a review of escape rooms in nursing education during her graduate coursework. She is a Clinical Educator at Boone Health in Columbia, Missouri, where she primarily works with graduate and new-to-practice nurses. She is the Nurse Residency Program Director for Boone Health and oversaw the program's journey to ANCC PTAP accreditation. She enjoys supporting nurses entering the profession and incorporating new technology and simulation into her teaching.

Kimberly Reschke, DNP, APRN is a graduate of Resurrection University (Bachelor of Science in Nursing) and Rush University (Doctor of Nursing Practice). She has served as a clinical assistant professor in the Loyola University Chicago, Marcella Niehoff School of Nursing since 2022. She uses engaging, interactive, and meaningful pedagogical strategies to facilitate learning and engage students in the classroom to improve student understanding, retention, and application of pathophysiology concepts. Her research has focused on translating current best evidence with informatics knowledge to improve follow-up appointment completion rates and identify barriers to reduce hospital readmission rates by using computerized clinical information systems. By analyzing the data collected from computerized clinical information systems, she can better understand the causes of readmission and develop strategies to reduce them. This includes developing protocols for follow-up appointments, creating systems for tracking patient progress, and providing education for patients and their families.

Miranda Smith, EdD, AGACNP-BC is a Clinical Assistant Professor at the University of Alabama in Huntsville College of Nursing. She has been teaching since 2004 in clinical, classroom, simulation, and online learning environments. She teaches critical care nursing in the prelicensure BSN program, multiple courses within the accelerated program, RN-BSN/dual programs, and chairs DNP students and serves on PhD dissertation committees. Her research interests include the transition of nursing students as they grow into their professional roles, innovative teaching-learning strategies, and the use of technology in and outside the classroom to enhance clinical judgment. She earned her ADN from Wallace State Community College in 2002, her BSN from the University of North Alabama (UNA) in 2012, and her MSN in nursing education from UNA. She earned her EdD in Instructional Leadership in 2021 from the University of Alabama. She received her MSN as an adult gerontological acute care nurse practitioner in December 2023.

Joni Tornwall, PhD, RN, ANEF is an Associate Clinical Professor in the College of Nursing at The Ohio State University. She is also Codirector of the Academy for Teaching Innovation, Excellence, and Scholarship and Director of Assessment and Evaluation in the College of Nursing. She began her nursing career as an RN circulator and surgical technologist in the operating room. She later transitioned to staff positions in adult education, ultimately earning her PhD in Education dedicating her full-time work to academic nursing education. She has over 20 years of experience in teaching online and face-to-face courses at the undergraduate and graduate levels in academic success, scholarly writing for DNPs, instructional design for nurses, EBP, and professional and interprofessional concepts in nursing. Her research is focused on nursing education, and her primary areas of interest are innovative strategies in teaching and learning in the health professions and student-to-student peer review and feedback. She is a fellow in the NLN Academy of Nursing Education, served as a Fulbright Specialist in Finland in 2023, and she has won the College of Nursing Outstanding Faculty Colleague Award multiple times. She serves on the editorial board of two nursing education journals and interviews innovators in nursing education for broadly distributed podcasts. Her record of publications and presentations reflects her investment in innovative learning design and health professions education in collaboration with local, national, and international nurse-faculty colleagues and academic-practice organizations.

Yeyin Yi, DNP, APRN is a Clinical Assistant Professor who joined Loyola University Chicago Marcella Niehoff School of Nursing in 2018. She primarily teaches online prelicensure nursing core curriculum of pathophysiology, pharmacology, health assessment, and nursing fundamentals. She received the Illinois Board of Higher Education Nurse Educator Fellowship dedicated to quality and innovative teaching in 2022 and has been nominated for awards recognizing excellence in teaching, student engagement, and global awareness. Her area of scholarship involves the integration of contextualized real-world clinical application in an academic framework focused on holistic inclusion of mental health and education efficacy and translational application of evidence-based nursing practice. She is a board-certified adult-gerontology acute care nurse practitioner with clinical experience traversing trauma/surgical critical care, postacute rehabilitation, and primary gerontological practice. She thoroughly enjoys spending time and creating memories with her cherished family, which includes her beloved daughters, supportive husband, encouraging parents, and treasured sister and extended family.

Christine Zimmerman, PhD, RN, CHSE is an Assistant Clinical Professor at the University of Missouri–Kansas City School of Nursing and Health Studies. She has taught in a variety of undergraduate courses and graduate simulation courses. As the Director of Clinical Simulation her practice involves the creation, implementation, and evaluation of high-fidelity simulation scenarios, including escape rooms, for the undergraduate and graduate nursing programs.

Foreword

Imagine trying to care for a patient who is entombed in a metal tube that has only a few access holes for providing physical care and assessments. These were constraints placed on nurses when an innovative technology, the iron lung, was used to support breathing for patients with polio through much of the 1940s and 1950s. A vicious epidemic and new technologies required nurses to rethink and reshape their approach to care. Sound familiar? The modern-day COVID-19 pandemic similarly forced nurses, nurse leaders, and nurse educators to rethink how they delivered care in a state of emergency while also rapidly rethinking technology-dependent educational delivery.

During polio's peak impact, the National League for Nursing (NLN) was a leader in shaping care delivery and helping integrate technology and innovative care approaches into nursing practice. That tradition continues with this text. On the heels of the COVID-19 pandemic and an explosion in technology for teaching and practice, the NLN and the editors have gathered expert insight into current and future readiness. Educators eager to try something new, to better use technologies they have today, or to forge a future-proofed skill set will all find something of value in this work. No matter your rationale, you are probably well aware that technology is now one of the biggest influences on educational delivery and success. It holds the greatest potential for satisfying the needs of the growing diversity of learners seeking nursing as a profession, meeting the pressure on academia to prepare an even more technologically and practice-ready workforce faster than ever before, and bridging the gaps of high-value clinical sites for students.

Educational technology has matured to the point where we can indeed achieve our highest educational aspirations for teaching and learning. The book and the work of its editors and contributors clearly reflect the NLN's continued leadership and guidance in achieving such educational excellence. The chapters of this work are a collection of personal insights, the latest evidence, experience-tested tricks of the trade, and technologies that promise to maintain joy in teaching along with student enthusiasm for learning. The ideas within will open doors, eyes, hearts, and minds to the many new and exciting ways that technology can support teaching and learning.

Technology has helped to make incredible strides in extending the length and quality of life for patients and in increasing the boundaries of traditional site-based care. It can similarly break down the boundaries of a traditional classroom by diversifying the ways in which we plan, assess, and deliver engaging and impactful educational experiences. With fewer boundaries, we can invite a larger and more diverse group of future nurses into a path toward preparation. As educators, we have technologies today that hold incredible potential for high-impact learning that were not conceivable even a few years ago. We must maximize the power of current and emerging technologies to prepare a highly knowledgeable and skilled workforce that is ready to heal our ailing health care system.

Matthew Byrne, PhD, RN, CNE
Nurse Administrator
Mayo Clinic
Rochester, Minnesota

Preface

The COVID-19 pandemic, which began in the United States in 2020, was the catalyst for a rapid shift in nursing education, moving classroom-based education to online formats. However, many faculty did not know how to pivot, and they asked the National League for Nursing (NLN) for help. To address this need, the NLN created a resource center of COVID-19 tips and resources for educators. A small team from the NLN Division for Innovation in Education Excellence, with contributions from NLN Simulation leaders, including myself, compiled virtual resources for educators to integrate into their programs. This robust list of resources also included how-to examples, a much needed extra step to help overwhelmed educators (https://www.nln.org/education/coronavirus-resource-center#webinar). These resources are free and can be shared widely with nursing educators across the country.

As a follow-up, the team hosted a series of Taking Aim webinars to address online teaching challenges and success stories. These webinars focused on how to address the cognitive, psychomotor, and affective domains of learning. Similar resources were shared through the NLN Nursing Edge blog and podcast series.

I was introduced to Andrew in 2020 when I served as a moderator for his NLN webinar, "Taking Aim at Good Teaching: Assessing for Learning in the Classroom." Andrew introduced the concept of gamification as a tool for checking students' understanding of concepts and for engaging learners. The success of that webinar led to the two of us conducting a workshop at the 2021 NLN Education Summit, during which we walked through the what and how of using technology to engage and evaluate learners. Leading by example, we introduced several learning tools, many incorporating gamification elements. The tools simulated real-world opportunities for attendees to apply to their own teaching.

Andrew and I have continued to work together in a variety of NLN courses and projects, and this partnership—that of a nurse educator and an instructional technologist who are both passionate about teaching with technology—led to the development and publication of *Teaching Tomorrow's Nurses: A Technology-Enhanced Approach*.

We hope you will use this book to situate yourself in the why behind how technology can successfully be used in the classroom, both in person and online, and then jump in, learn about an innovative technology tool, and try it out in the classroom using examples provided. We cannot promise that it will be a perfect teaching moment, but we can promise that technology will help support your teaching and—more importantly—your learners. Have fun!

Jennifer O'Rourke, PhD, APRN, CHSE
Andrew Bobal, EdD

Acknowledgments

We would like to thank the National League for Nursing for supporting our commitment to promoting best practices in nursing education and technology. A special thank you to Dr. Susan Forneris, who mentored us in our roles as consultants for the NLN, and Dr. Barbara Patterson, who connected us in our mutual love of technology.

Jennifer O'Rourke, PhD, APRN, CHSE
Andrew Bobal, EdD

Contents

List of Figures, Tables, and Boxes

LIST OF BOXES

Transformative Nursing Education: Harnessing Technology for Enhanced Learning and Practice

Joni Tornwall, PhD, RN, ANEF

Academic nurse educators have historically been early adopters of technology for teaching and learning. Several factors drive trends in adoption of learning technology in nursing education, including a strong sense of value for innovation in nursing, a desire to engage and retain increasingly diverse learners, and a requirement for nursing education to prepare graduates with skills aligned with rapid advances in health care technology. Global and societal factors, such as the COVID-19 pandemic in 2020, have accelerated the rate of technology adoption in nursing education, and this trend in responding to global events in health care and education with increased use of technology is expected to continue (Wolters Kluwer & National League for Nursing, 2021). Furthermore, broader and deeper integration of technology in nursing education pressures nurse educators to contribute to the literature in sound pedagogical practices that optimize the student's learning experience (Poindexter, 2021). However, complex barriers hinder educators' efforts to use evidence-based educational approaches to embed advanced learning technology in optimal ways throughout the nursing curriculum.

Swiftly evolving academic and health care landscapes make it difficult for instructors to choose from a vast array of available technologies. A shrinking nurse-educator workforce and increasing faculty workloads reduce available time to learn how to use technology and implement it effectively in the various types of spaces where nursing education takes place (Smart et al., 2020; Wolters Kluwer, 2021). Essential questions arise from concerns about how the nursing discipline can balance the demand for a greater quantity and quality of technology-enhanced learning with challenges to feasibility in implementation. How will nurse educators respond to pressure to use more complex technology in the classroom while dealing with constraints on funding, privacy and security concerns, the transition from task-based to concept-based curricula and competency-based education, and their own lack of time and professional development resources for learning how to use new technologies?

This chapter provides a broad overview of the importance of technology in nursing education and how the nursing discipline situates learning technology as a key component in the educational process. It describes conceptual and practical ways nurse educators can grapple with selection and implementation of learning technology tools and foreshadows future trends in learning technology. It proposes a schema based on 10 fundamental factors for approaching broad questions about integration of educational technology in nursing curricula. This chapter aims to help educators disentangle a dynamic multitude of options and opportunities in educational technology and develop effective solutions to specific problems in teaching and learning.

THE ROLE OF TECHNOLOGY IN NURSING EDUCATION

Nursing education is undergoing a transformation in paradigm and process. Research has revealed a steady decline in competency of nursing students at the end of their academic programs over the past decade (Kavanagh & Sharpnack, 2021). In response to these findings, leaders and innovators in nursing education are working to understand how technology can support a transformation in the process to reverse negative trends in the competency of graduates. The body of evidence has shown that embedded technology supports positive learning outcomes for students through more realistic simulation (Harerimana & Mtshali, 2020), universal learning design and access that is inclusive of all learners (Lucas et al., 2022), and preparation to use technology graduates will encounter in the workplace (e.g., informatics, telehealth, patient monitors). Technology promises to support clinical reasoning and decision-making through artificial intelligence (AI) (De Gagne, 2023), analyze large amounts of data to predict student success and provide early warnings for at-risk students (Pelletier et al., 2023), and provide multiple opportunities to practice applied nursing concepts and demonstrate competency in increasingly authentic virtual environments (De Gagne et al., 2023).

Nurse educators acknowledge the potential in learning technology to provide nursing students with diverse and repeatable opportunities for practice and application of content in authentic health care contexts and reflect on rationales for clinical decisions (Patterson & Forneris, 2023). They recognize that students, the direct-care nurses of the future, need preparation to be subject-matter experts in selection and implementation of technology in health care practice (Freeman & Wilson, 2023). However, gaps in skills and knowledge of nurse educators to embed technology in nursing curricula call for more intense professional development efforts in an academic environment where instructors' time is already stretched to the limit (National Advisory Council on Nurse Education and Practice, 2021).

How do these pedagogical goals related to technology in nursing education operationalize into practical and effective instructional designs and learning technology tool implementations? The first step is to clarify how current learning technology tools support student achievement of nursing competencies. The next step is to look toward creating a future educational environment in which more advanced learning technology contributes in meaningful ways to development of every student as a competent, practice-ready nursing graduate.

CURRENT LEARNING TECHNOLOGY IN NURSING EDUCATION

Some familiar learning technology tools will continue to evolve along with transformative innovation in higher education and nursing toward creation of progressively more authentic and interactive learning environments.

Learning Management Systems

Learning management systems (LMSs) have expanded access to education for learners who are widely dispersed and have demanding work and personal lives. LMSs make course content available and interaction with instructors and peers possible anytime and anywhere there is a connection to the internet. LMSs that stand the test of educational transformation will need to capitalize on the power of AI; provide high-fidelity interaction between students and course content, peers, and instructor; use data analytics to support assessment and evaluation; and integrate adaptive, personalized learning for every student.

Web- and Videoconferencing Platforms

Web- and videoconferencing platforms surged in use during the COVID-19 pandemic and secured a solid role in the future of nursing education and health care. Education across a broad spectrum of didactic, clinical, and lab settings is supported by webconferencing tools. They support a wide range of teaching and learning activities, including lectures, informal student group meetings, objective structured clinical exams, virtual clinical experiences, and telehealth training. Watch for webconferencing tools to evolve into increasingly more immersive applications that make interaction between remote individuals feel more like face-to-face, in-person learning, gradually becoming more like a three-dimensional virtual reality (VR) environment known as the metaverse (De Gagne, 2023).

Eportfolios

Eportfolios and other strategies for comprehensive assessment of individual students over the course of their program have gained popularity over recent years. Eportfolios and similar tools allow students to create a showcase of different types of evidence of their academic achievements throughout their academic programs, provide opportunities for academic staff to assess competency development at individual and program levels, and serve as digital augmentation to traditional resumes for potential employers as they consider hiring decisions. As educational institutions face growing pressure to meet regulatory requirements, document student learning outcomes, and make postgraduate job placement information visible, expect use of applications and tools for comprehensive competency assessment of individual students to increase and be referred to in more general terms, such as competency tracking tools. As competency-based education gains a stronghold in nursing and assessment standards lean more toward holistic evaluation of competencies based on multiple sources of data, nursing programs will need a means for students to create, collect, and display evidence of their attainment of professional nursing competencies (American Association of Colleges of Nursing, 2021, 2023).

FUTURE TRENDS IN LEARNING TECHNOLOGY

Although we do not have a clear picture of how learning technologies will evolve and be situated in higher education, certain technological innovations in teaching and learning are emerging as key influences that will shape the future of nursing education.

Virtual and Augmented Reality

VR and augmented reality, referred to under the umbrella term extended reality (XR), promise to transform immersive experiences in clinical and classroom learning into progressively more authentic and intense encounters than students have experienced in the past. XR environments allow participants to interact in real time with others (or avatar-like representations of others) in the same physical space. Participants can share virtual whiteboards, presentations, three-dimensional models (e.g., medical equipment), and procedural demonstrations and interact with simulated patients or manikins present in the same physical space as the learner. Participants can observe the physical location and actions of colleagues and patients in a virtual room and even observe authentic affect and emotional responses of others. Possibilities for application of XR in the nursing education classroom are seemingly infinite, but the effect of XR on learning is not yet clearly understood (Ryan et al., 2022). There will be an urgent need for educational research exploring the effectiveness of instruction in XR environments for many years to come.

Machine Learning and Artificial Intelligence

Machine learning and AI are also generating excitement as well as some trepidation in nursing education. There is substantial potential for AI, alone or in combination with other technologies, to create more realistic simulations, analyze data to generate early warnings for at-risk students, recognize patterns in learning and adapt instruction to individual student needs, and lighten the workload of overextended faculty. At the same time, concerns related to faculty training in AI, student privacy, academic integrity, and clarity regarding how students should be trained to use AI in nursing practice present barriers to rapid adoption and integration of AI in nursing education (De Gagne, 2023).

Digital Hardware and Software

Digital hardware and software have allowed students to produce multimedia as evidence of their learning for many years. In the future, software applications that allow more complex creative expression and course content creation by students are expected to expand in number and capability and take on a more important role in nursing education (Pelletier et al., 2023). The nursing discipline already requires professional nurses to create evidence-based presentations and education for patients and health care administrators, communicate through multimedia in virtual environments, and innovate using the latest technology. Nurse educators will need to enhance their efforts to advance student skills beyond traditional presentation tools and video creation to move progressively toward interprofessional collaboration on unique, innovative products such as new applications for use in health care, evidence-based algorithms for clinical decision support, and resources for patients to care for themselves outside of a hospital. These types of innovations are possible only if nurse educators prepare their students to understand how and when to use emerging technologies, such as AI and low-/no-code technologies (MacLean, 2021).

PRACTICAL APPROACHES TO BROAD QUESTIONS

Radical, rapid, and sudden change is common in health care and nursing education, and the understanding of cognitive processes underpinning how humans learn is also evolving. The body of evidence about the effects of learning technologies on student learning outcomes is currently based primarily on student satisfaction and self-assessments of their own learning, which can be inaccurate (Lee et al., 2022). Nursing education research based on cognitive science and conceptual models of teaching and learning produces stronger evidence of the complex effects of technology on student learning (Onello & Moulton, 2021). A shift in the underpinnings of nursing education research to evidence-based neurocognitive principles and learning theory in combination with innovative approaches to teaching will build a stronger body of literature.

Pragmatic, evidence-based, enduring approaches to implementation of technology in nursing education will help nurse educators create engaging and flexible instruction that evolves with the changes in a dynamic technology landscape (Kavanagh & Sharpnack, 2021). Algorithms for selecting technology, weaving it seamlessly into the instructional process, implementing it in real-world, authentic learning environments, and evaluating its effectiveness can be derived from a strong body of empirical evidence combined with an innovative disposition toward technology in teaching.

An instructional design framework helps ensure that selected technology supports instructional goals (and avoids instructional strategies that end up supporting technology) and facilitates instructional decisions about how and when to use learning technology. The backward design framework (Wiggins & McTighe, 1998) provides a simple process for decision-making. Three key questions in backward design that should be asked before selecting any learning technology include the following: (1) What is the competency students need to achieve, or what is the specific, observable, measurable learning objective students need to demonstrate? (2) What would an assessment of student achievement of the competency or learning objective require them to do to show they have achieved the competency or objective? (3) What learning activities will students do to build skills, knowledge, and attitudes necessary to develop competence and do well on the assessment?

With the answers to these three questions in mind — the explicitly stated competency or objective, the observable assessment evidence of achievement, and the specific activity students need to engage in to develop proficiency — educators must then ask the essential question in selecting and evaluating technology: What types of technologies align well with the instructional purpose and support achievement of competencies and objectives, successful student performance on assessments, and student activities that produce meaningful learning?

TEN TIPS FOR SELECTING LEARNING TECHNOLOGY TOOLS

To answer this fundamental question about which type of technology is the best fit for an instructional purpose, educators can explore 10 facets in a broad decision framework for selection, implementation, and evaluation of learning technologies. Use this framework as you read this book to consider how each theory, concept, and learning technology applies to your teaching context. Consider these suggestions as you deal with new technologies that entice (or require) you to use them in your teaching and learning practice.

Align Technology With Broad Competencies and Learning Objectives

This is a fundamental principle in choosing learning technology. All other decisions about learning technology are second in priority to sound instructional design and alignment of technology with instructional purpose, and the backward design framework provides an easy-to-use three-phase model for achieving this alignment:

▶ Objective: Establish a clear instructional purpose with a direct connection to student achievement of a competency or learning objective.

▶ Assessment: Explicitly delineate what students need to do to demonstrate achievement of the competency or objective. What role will technology play in this demonstration?

▶ Activity: Describe how students will develop proficiency at the required level for success on the assessment. How does technology support student activities and self-assessment opportunities that lead to competency?

What to avoid: Avoid choosing technology based on interest, fun, availability, or popularity without first considering fundamental questions of instructional purpose and design.

Prioritize Selection of Institutionally Supported Learning Technology

Institutions are forced by external factors to create a balanced set of technology tools within their budget and ability to provide infrastructure support (Smart et al., 2020). Your choices in learning technology may be partially limited by the set of tools your organization provides. Even if choices are not restricted by institutional resources, consider institutionally supported tools first in your technology evaluation and selection. The advantages of using an institutionally supported tool are lower cost, availability of technical support, and likelihood of learner familiarity with the tool.

What to avoid: Avoid selecting a tool that has no institutional support. You or your learners may ultimately bear the cost for full access to the tool, and you, the instructor, will end up providing much of the technical support for your students as well as for yourself.

Find a Way to Measure the Value the Tool Adds to Learning

Collect data on student activity and experience associated with the tool. Ensure that data connect use of the tool with student learning outcomes that provide information about student experience with the tool (e.g., student satisfaction and self-perceptions of learning are important measures but do not provide complete assessment data) and, more importantly, evidence of student achievement of objectives and competencies related to the tool. How do you know students achieved the intended learning outcomes (grades provide only partial evidence of student achievement), and how do you know the technology tool supported student achievement? Evidence of attainment of observable, measurable learning outcomes in combination with data on student experience with a tool shows you, your students, and all others who are invested in nursing education that the tool has an important role (or not) in overall student outcomes and its use should be continued (or discontinued).

What to avoid: Avoid allowing time to pass during which a tool is used but no data are intentionally collected to demonstrate the tool's effectiveness. Those who support use of the tool will eventually want to know the return on their investment of resources.

Design a Data Collection Plan Based on Conceptual Models to Determine What Role, if Any, a Tool Played in Student Achievement of Learning Outcomes

Objective data on student achievement and subjective data on student and faculty experience with a tool over time should be used to make evidence-based decisions about which tools and technologies to keep and which to discontinue. Collection of these types of data requires planning before instruction begins, not after instruction occurs. Conceptualize the student learning experience using theoretical models and frameworks to explain how students learn using technology (Nes et al., 2021), and share your findings with colleagues through publications and presentations.

What to avoid: Avoid neglecting to design a data collection plan at the time instruction is being designed, or collecting data but not taking time to find out what it reveals about how learning technology contributed to student learning. You and everyone who is invested in nursing education will want to know the rationale and story behind your effective teaching practices and the role technology played in student success.

Consider Accessibility, Potential for Bias, and Data Privacy and Security

Laws, technology standards, and educational regulations require learning technology used in instruction to be accessible by individuals with disabilities and secure enough to protect student privacy. Institutionally supported tools are often vetted and pre-determined to meet accessibility and security requirements, but it is the instructor's responsibility to know whether this is true or not and take measures to ensure student access, safety, and data privacy in the use of learning technology. The burden of recognizing potential to introduce bias through learning technology (e.g., bias in AI algorithms, socioeconomic factors affecting access, or interaction bias in collaboration tools) also falls on the instructor. No tool is completely accessible, free of potential for bias, and totally secure. The essential questions are, To what degree is the tool accessible, bias free, and secure? and How will potential breeches related to the tool be mitigated?

What to avoid: Avoid selecting a tool that has not been vetted against standards of accessibility, security, and potential for bias, or failing to compare the relative risks inherent in a tool to the relative benefits to learning.

Know Your Own Tolerance for Risk

Although the first five considerations may seem to draw restrictive parameters around innovation, creativity with new tools and original approaches to learning are still quite feasible. Rather than thinking of the cautions listed earlier as contributing to anxiety about using learning technology, think of them as measures on a continuum of risk versus benefit. Determine where your personal tolerance for risk falls on the risk-benefit spectrum specific to a particular learning technology tool. Know that your tolerance for risk will be different for every tool and different from your colleagues' risk tolerance, so assess each tool independently and choose those that promise to provide, as you see it, the most benefit to learning and the least risk in terms of user experience, investment of resources, and your teaching effectiveness.

What to avoid: Avoid implementing a high-risk, low-reward tool or implementing a high-risk, high-reward tool when your tolerance (or your students' tolerance) is low for technical challenges and lack of support.

Assess the Digital Readiness of Students

Educators generally recognize that most students enter higher education with at least some technical savvy that is often related to mobile devices and social networks and less frequently associated with academic and scholarly goals (Smart et al., 2020). It is difficult to determine learner readiness for use of educational technology in advance of tool selection, but a broad characterization of student groups based on demographics, socioeconomic factors, health care experience, previous academic experience, and other relevant factors can help you select technology that is a good fit for learners. For example, keeping your instructional purpose and learner audience in mind simultaneously, the technology you choose to teach the same content for a nursing program at an R1 research institution, a community college, or an institution in a foreign country may be different for each setting.

What to avoid: Avoid assuming the same educational content can be taught using the same technology without considering the learner context, including the general characteristics of the learners as a group. Remember to design instruction using the three steps of backward design; then, let learner characteristics and context work with the instructional purpose to determine your choice of technology.

Keep Your Eye on Technology Use in the Real World of Current Nursing Practice

It is imperative that nurse educators prepare students to use and evaluate technology they will encounter in health care practice. Advances in decision-making support for health care professionals require critical judgments about the validity of digitally generated recommendations for patient care. Advances in informatics in health care require nurses to understand the underlying data and the applications used to manipulate them. Advances in medical procedures and equipment that nurses and patients are expected to use require training to protect health care quality and patient safety. It is almost impossible to prepare nursing students with all skills and knowledge they will need to use technology in practice, but it is feasible to prepare students to be digitally literate lifelong learners who thrive in technology-infused health care environments.

What to avoid: Avoid inattention to advances in the world of health care practice. Stay in touch with common and specialized health care settings according to the courses you teach. Stay aware of technology trends affecting how health care is delivered in those settings. Ensure good alignment between the learning technology students use in their education and how they will use technology in common and specialized practice settings (Nes et al., 2021; Smart et al., 2020).

Anticipate Change

Every tool you adopt will eventually undergo updates, redesigns, changes in commercial ownership, or ultimately be phased out and replaced by another more advanced tool that addresses contemporary learner needs. Consider how you will handle the transition of content and instructional processes from one tool to another as you select any new technology. Generally, creating or uploading content in a new tool and spending time and effort to design a smooth learner experience within the tool involve a significant investment of time and resources for an educator. When that tool is eventually phased out, what amount of effort and resources will be required to transfer the existing content and instruction to a new tool?

What to avoid: Avoid selecting a technology tool that requires a significant amount of time and effort to input content but provides no way to export content in common file formats for transfer into another tool.

Anticipate Global Events That Impact the Use of Technology

A pandemic that would force nursing education to move rapidly to a virtual environment seemed unimaginable in 2019. After the COVID-19 pandemic, hindsight showed that nurse educators can respond successfully to disruptive global events with innovation and resilience (Altmiller & Pepe, 2022). How much stronger could the response to future global events be if nurse educators anticipate the next disruptive event before it happens? Predicting specific scenarios is not as important as preparing to flex rapidly in response to interruptions in the usual way nursing education is delivered. Imagine, for example, the improbable event that the digital infrastructure supporting nurse education fails, and broad access to the internet stops for students. How will you prepare for broad and sudden failure or removal of access to the technology your teaching depends on?

What to avoid: Avoid assuming that technology and the infrastructure it is built on will not fail. Academic nursing created an educational environment in which face-to-face learning can be replaced largely by virtual opportunities. In doing so, we created a nursing education paradigm largely dependent on connectivity in a digital environment plagued by threats to cybersecurity. What will you do if students lose access to the technology and infrastructure that connects them to the nursing education we provide?

CONCLUSION

Learning technology plays a profoundly important role in nursing education. It connects diverse groups of learners and faculty in shared collaboration spaces. Learning technology adapts content to fit the unique needs of individual learners and prepares students to use health care technology they will encounter in nursing practice. Technology-based simulations are transforming the way future nurses learn to make competent clinical decisions and provide high-quality, safe patient care. Opportunities to practice skills, rehearse knowledge, and apply concepts in different scenarios are progressively growing in similarity to the real world as AI and XR emerge as potentially powerful influences in nursing education.

Learning technology integration in nursing education is projected to increase in breadth and depth in the future. Selection, implementation, and evaluation of the effectiveness of learning technology in supporting student achievement of learning outcomes should always be underpinned by sound pedagogy and strong instructional design. Technology augments good teaching but it will not replace skilled nurse educators who understand innovation in teaching, human cognition, and complex learning challenges. Moreover, nursing students must develop broad evaluative judgment related to technology, especially AI, to recognize the value it adds as well as its potential risks to quality and safety. Competency achievement for graduating nurses begins with innovative nurse educators willing to take measured risks in learning environments that are grounded in rigorous research evidence and, at the same time, stretching conventional approaches to teaching with technology.

References

Altmiller, G., & Pepe, L. H. (2022). Influence of technology in supporting quality and safety in nursing education. *Nursing Clinics of North America, 57*(4), 551–562. https://doi.org/10.1016/j.cnur.2022.06.005

American Association of Colleges of Nursing (AACN). (2021). *The essentials: Core competencies for professional nursing education*. https://www.aacnnursing.org/Education-Resources/AACN-Essentials

American Association of Colleges of Nursing (AACN). (2023). *Guiding principles for competency-based education and assessment*. https://www.aacnnursing.org/Portals/

0/PDFs/Essentials/Guiding-Principles-for-CBE-Assessment.pdf

De Gagne, J. C. (2023). The state of artificial intelligence in nursing education: Past, present, and future directions. *International Journal of Environmental Research and Public Health*, 20(6), 4884. https://doi.org/10.3390/ijerph20064884

De Gagne, J. C., Randall, P. S., Rushton, S., Park, H. K., Cho, E., Yamane, S. S., & Jung, D. (2023). The use of metaverse in nursing education: An umbrella review. *Nurse Educator*, 48(3), E73–E78. https://doi.org/10.1097/NNE.0000000000001327.

Freeman, R., & Wilson, M. (2023). Starting at the top: Developing an informatics-competent and capable nursing workforce. *Nursing Management*, 54(5), 6–10. https://doi.org/10.1097/nmg.0000000000000016

Harerimana, A., & Mtshali, N. G. (2020). Using exploratory and confirmatory factor analysis to understand the role of technology in nursing education. *Nurse Education Today*, 92, 104490. https://doi.org/10.1016/j.nedt.2020.104490

Kavanagh, J. M., & Sharpnack, P. A. (2021). Crisis in competency: A defining moment in nursing education. *Online Journal of Issues in Nursing*, 26(1). https://doi.org/10.3912/OJIN.Vol26No01Man02

Lee, A. S. D., Owings, C. R., Johnson, J. M., & Carruth, M. S. (2022). Brain science-based innovative collaborative teaching to facilitate nursing education. *Journal of Nursing Education*, 61(3), 162–166. https://doi.org/10.3928/01484834-20211128-08

Lucas, L. S., Silbert-Flagg, J., & D'Aoust, R. F. (2022). Nursing students with disabilities: A guide to providing accommodations. *Nursing Clinics of North America*, 57(4), 671–683. https://doi.org/10.1016/j.cnur.2022.06.012

MacLean, A. (2021). Software development trends 2021. *Canadian Journal of Nursing Informatics*, 16(1). https://www.proquest.com/docview/2561882986

National Advisory Council on Nurse Education and Practice (NACNEP). (2021). *Preparing nurse faculty and addressing the shortage of nurse faculty and clinical preceptors (No. 17)*. https://www.hrsa.gov/sites/default/files/hrsa/advisory-committees/nursing/reports/nacnep-17report-2021.pdf

Nes, A. A. G., Steindal, S. A., Larsen, M. H., Heer, H. C., Lærum-Onsager, E., & Gjevjon, E. R. (2021). Technological literacy in nursing education: A scoping review. *Journal of Professional Nursing*, 37(2), 320–334. https://doi.org/10.1016/j.profnurs.2021.01.008

Onello, R. L., & Moulton, M. C. (2021). From self-confidence to self-calibration: Using brain science to move the needle in nursing education. *Nursing Education Perspectives*, 42(3), 134–135. https://doi.org/10.1097/01.NEP.0000000000000818

Patterson, B., & Forneris, S. (2023). Moving beyond facts: It is time to rethink the practice of teaching. *Nursing Education Perspectives*, 44(3), 139. https://doi.org/10.1097/01.NEP.0000000000001133

Pelletier, K., Robert, J., Muscanell, N., McCormack, M., Reeves, J., Arbino, N., & Grajek, S. (2023). *2023 EDUCAUSE horizon report: Teaching and learning edition*. EDUCAUSE. https://www.educause.edu/horizon-report-teaching-and-learning-2023

Poindexter, K. (2021). The future of nursing education: Reimagined. *Nursing Education Perspectives*, 42(6), 335–336. https://doi.org/10.1097/01.NEP.0000000000000907

Ryan, G. V., Callaghan, S., Rafferty, A., Higgins, M. F., Mangina, E., & McAuliffe, F. (2022). Learning outcomes of immersive technologies in health care student education: Systematic review of the literature. *Journal of Medical Internet Research*, 24(2), e30082. https://doi.org/10.2196/30082

Smart, D., Ross, K., Carollo, S., & Williams-Gilbert, W. (2020). Contextualizing instructional technology to the demands of nursing education. *CIN: Computers, Informatics, Nursing*, 38(1), 18–27. https://doi.org/10.1097/CIN.0000000000000565

Wiggins, G., & McTighe, J. (1998). Backward design. In *Understanding by design* (pp. 13–34). Association for Supervision and Curriculum Development.

Wolters Kluwer & National League for Nursing. (2021). *Forecast for the future: Technology trends in nursing education*. https://www.wolterskluwer.com/en/solutions/lippincott-nursing-faculty/dean-survey

2

Pedagogical Considerations When Teaching With Technology

Michelle C. Moulton, DNP, RN, CHSE, CNE
Rachel Onello, PhD, RN, CHSE, CNE, CNE-cl, CNL, ANEF

"Technology is anything that wasn't around when you were born."
—Alan Kay (computer scientist)

"Any sufficiently advanced technology is equivalent to magic."
—Arthur C. Clarke (author)

For many of us, these two quotes capture the definition and presence of technology in our daily lives. The first quote is seemingly obvious and the second a bit more whimsical, but both capture the novelty, rapid pace, and sometimes mysterious characteristics of technology. The daily average amount of time people spend using the internet is approximately 7 hours — nearly equal to the amount of time spent sleeping (Kemp, 2023). There is little question about the central role technology plays in people's lives, work, and leisure.

LET PEDAGOGY BE THE DRIVER

The extensive use of technology in educational settings mirrors that of our professional and personal lives and continues to grow. There is no shortage of technology-enhanced teaching tools available. The endless different ways to use technology to support education, at any level, can create more of a dilemma than a solution for educators. The burden rests on educators to align expertise in teaching pedagogy with the best modality to promote discovery and transformation. Using technology to support, extend, or propel the learning process must not be an afterthought but an intentional and informed integration of evidence, strategy, and tools that enhance, rather than hinder, the outcome. Yet, nurse educators find themselves responding to the pressures of adopting technology quickly and diffusely. Allowing technology to drive teaching strategies and decisions, rather than pedagogical principles and learning outcomes, narrows the educational experience to focus on the mechanical delivery of teaching rather than the transformational process of learning. When technology is advocated as a tool to build

13

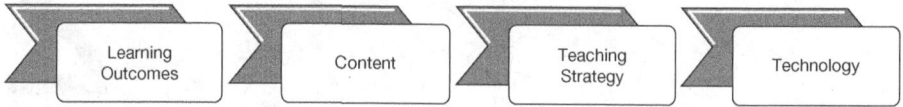

FIGURE 2.1 Outline of Process to Align Learning Outcomes With Effective Teaching Strategies.

an integrated and engaging learning experience, educators can guide learners toward mastery. Figure 2.1 outlines a simple process nurse educators can use to help align the learning outcomes with the most effective teaching strategy and technology application that promotes competency development.

Sound educational pedagogy begins with identifying the desired learning outcomes that stem from the educational experience goals. Beginning with the end in mind serves as an anchor from which every pedagogical decision derives, informing the delivery and format of the learning experience. The second step, content, reflects the selection of topic areas informed by the practice of nursing and health care delivery. Inexperienced educators may fall into the trap of allowing content or practice trends to inform educational experiences without first being tied to the learning outcomes. The temptation to begin with content is often driven by the pressure educators experience related to ensuring that learners have the right knowledge and skills to function in the practice setting. While this is a worthwhile endeavor, a heavy focus on teaching nursing practice knowledge and skills acontextually and without a clear, objective, and shared mental model on what practice looks like creates vast variability in the observable performance measures of the new graduate upon entry into practice (Forneris et al., 2022). Once the learning outcomes are linked to practice-informed content areas, teaching strategies can be selected that mirror the directive of the goal. For example, if the learning outcome is to apply content knowledge, then a learning activity designed to use existing knowledge to solve a presented problem, such as a case study, promotes the application of knowledge to make clinical decisions to address embedded problems in the case study. The final step is to determine the best technology to support the delivery of the teaching strategy. Using the case study example, uncovering the patient care needs outlined in the case may require the use of an electronic health record to determine the nursing care decisions required of the exercise.

Figure 2.2 adds context to the process that supports nurse educators' call to design learning experiences enhanced with technology. Learning outcomes define the achievement of knowledge, skills, or abilities, but a commitment to the clarity and assurance of systematically guiding learners toward meeting the outcomes requires a strategic, curricular, and programmatic shared mentality. There is a shift in nursing education toward using a competency-based education model that inspires academic-practice partnerships to cocreate a pathway toward competence and practice readiness (NLN Strategic Action Group, 2023). A competency-based education approach to teaching and learning may be new to nursing education, but it is not new to the pedagogy and science of learning. Early variations of competency-based education can be traced back several hundred years to apprenticeship and craft guild models of training, with leaders in K-12 education setting the stage for its use in contemporary higher education environments (Nodine, 2016).

Competency-based education shifts the focus from an emphasis on teaching toward an emphasis on learning (Barr & Tagg, 1995). The paradigm shift requires educators to

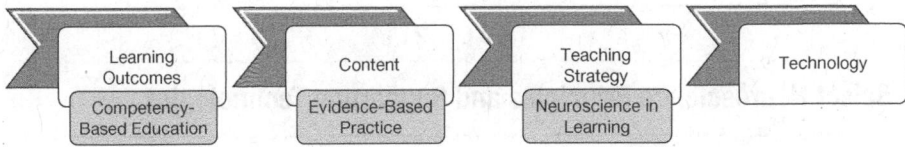

FIGURE 2.2 Context to the Process That Supports Design Learning With Technology.

guide learners along a continuum of milestones that mark their progress toward competence (Frank et al., 2010). Such a shift challenges educators to make radical and fundamental advancements in teaching strategies to include more formative, experiential, patient care–oriented learning encounters that more accurately reflect that of the practice environment. The thoughtful integration of technology with evidence-based teaching strategies provides the pathway for learners to progress from milestone to milestone. Additionally, technology can support the collection, analysis, and storage of data used to evaluate and measure learners' trajectory toward competence.

The emphasis on guiding learners toward building competence toward a clear and achievable measure of nursing practice provides clarity to the learning outcomes, strengthening the anchor from which learning experiences will be built. Underpinning the content selection is the rigor of using evidence-based practice to define and determine the specific practice-driven knowledge, skills, and abilities. When selecting the teaching strategy, the educator benefits from a strong understanding in neuroscience of learning principles that embolden learners to engage with the learning experience effectively and meaningfully. The selected technology to deliver the evidence-based teaching and learning strategy is inextricably linked to the desired goal and provides the vehicle to guide learners toward a clear, measurable mark of success.

A nurse educator's approach to thoughtful technology integration reciprocates with a solid understanding of the science of learning (i.e., the neuroscience of learning), which attempts to explain how learners learn. Understanding learning science provides a mental model from which to make pedagogical decisions (e.g., the design and delivery of learning experiences with technology). Additionally, a solid comprehension of neuroscience, combined with key theoretical concepts, provides a pedagogical foundation from which nurse educators can create opportunities for learners to apply knowledge to patient care experiences. It offers the type of contextual and transformative learning required of clinical practice.

Understanding neuroscience provides a mental model from which to make pedagogical decisions that involve designing and delivering technology-enhanced learning experiences that align with how the brain is wired to learn. Intentional and thoughtful use of technology can leverage neuroscience principles, leading to increased engagement with content. The more learners use content and access stored information, the more durable their learning (Carey, 2015). Technologies provide opportunities for learners to work with content, store information, construct new meaning, and encode information in meaningful ways that can be accessed readily from memory. Although not an exhaustive list, Table 2.1 provides an overview of select neuroscience principles and examples of technologies that are effective in leveraging brain engagement.

Figure 2.3 provides an example of how an educator might design an educational learning experience in which the learning outcome (e.g., Recognize salient cues...)

TABLE 2.1

Select Neuroscience Principles and Supporting Technologies

Neuroscience Principle	Description	Supporting Technologies
Priming	Formative pretesting (Carey, 2015); preexposure to information before explicit study enhances learning on subsequent exposure (Unger & Sloutsky, 2022)	➤ Audience polling ➤ Online audience engagement platform ➤ Computer-adaptive quizzing
Retrieval Practice	Active recall of information from memory (Carpenter et al., 2022)	➤ Video prompt and response platforms ➤ Formative activity apps ➤ Quizzing, polling, or audience engagement platforms
Dual Coding	Combining visual images and words in a meaningful way (Weinstein et al.; 2018)	➤ Storyboards, mind maps, or graphic organizers ➤ Infographic design software ➤ Online multimedia content boards or visual workspaces
Metacognition	Reflection on and awareness of one's thinking and learning (Carpenter et al., 2022)	➤ Video prompt and response platforms ➤ Formative activity apps[*] ➤ Quizzing, polling, or audience engagement platforms

drives the identification of content (care of clients with impaired oxygenation), which in turn determines the appropriate teaching strategy (case study) and neuroscience principles (retrieval practice and metacognition) to enable development of the desired competency. The educator selects a technology (online audience engagement platform) that will support and facilitate the evidence-based teaching and learning in alignment with the desired learning outcome.

Beginning with the learning outcomes in mind, educators can more thoughtfully integrate technology into the teaching and learning process. This is especially important in an academic landscape where options for easily accessible technology are abundant. In the example in Fig. 2.3, an online audience engagement platform was identified as the technology of choice. When considering technology alignment it is important to recognize that there is not a single correct answer for these decisions. In this example, multiple technologies would have effectively promoted retrieval practice and metacognition to achieve the learning outcome. Computer-adaptive quizzing, interactive educational gaming, or formative competition-style polling are meaningful and effective options for outcomes in the cognitive domain.

Considering the domains of the learning outcome (cognitive, psychomotor, or affective) is essential for aligning the most appropriate technology with the teaching strategy

Learning Outcomes	Content	Teaching Strategy & Neuroscience Principles	Technology
Recognize salient cues when caring for a client with an acute change in condition	Care of clients with impaired oxygenation	Case study incorporating retrieval practice and metacognition	Online audience engagement platform

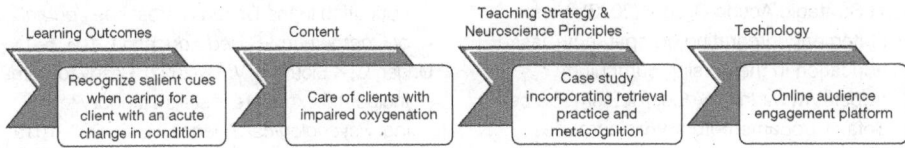

FIGURE 2.3 Example of an Educational Learning Experience.

and desired outcome. An educator may have access to a computer-adaptive quizzing application, a high-fidelity simulation manikin, or a virtual reality headset, but none of these experiences would serve as the most effective technology modality to learn a skill that requires the integration of many fine motor and cognitive steps to demonstrate mastery of a psychomotor competency. A task trainer with haptic feedback would be a more effective technology choice. Taking this example a step further, a learning outcome situated in the affective domain may require virtual reality to support the development of affective skills.

CONCLUSION

Nursing education continues its attentive response to calls to action that meet next-generation advancements for both academic and practice environments. A well-defined understanding of the role technology plays in enhancing learning experiences that reflect practice supports a renewed new graduate's trajectory toward competence and practice readiness. Nurse educators are well positioned to receive, design, and deliver neuroscience-inspired teaching strategies that use technology to meet the needs of the next-generation nursing workforce.

References

Barr, R. B., & Tagg, J. (1995). From teaching to learning—a new paradigm for undergraduate education. *Change: The Magazine of Higher Learning, 27*(6), 12–26. https://digitalcommons.unomaha.edu/slcehighered/60

Carey, B. (2015). *How we learn: The surprising truth about when, where, and why it happens.* Random House.

Carpenter, S. K., Pan, S. C., & Butler, A. C. (2022). The science of effective learning with spacing and retrieval practice. *Nature Reviews Psychology, 1,* 496–511. https://doi.org/10.1038/s44159-022-00089-1

Forneris, S. G., Tagliareni, E., & Allen, B. (2022). Accelerating to practice: Defining a competency-based education framework for nursing education Part 1.

Nursing Education Perspectives, 43(6), 363–367. https://api.semanticscholar.org/CorpusID:253187417

Frank, J. R., Snell, L. S., Cate, O. T., Holmboe, E. S., Carraccio, C., Swing, S. R., Harris, P., Glasgow, N. J., Campbell, C., Dath, D., Harden, R. M., Iobst, W., Long, D. M., Mungroo, R., Richardson, D. L., Sherbino, J., Silver, I., Taber, S., Talbot, M., & Harris, K. A. A. (2010). Competency-based medical education: Theory to practice. *Medical Teacher, 32*(8), 638–645. http://dx.doi.org/10.3109/0142159X.2010.501190

Kemp, S. (2023). Digital 2023 October global statshot report. Datareportal. https://datareportal.com/reports/digital-2023-october-global-statshot

NLN Strategic Action Group. (2023). Vision statement: Integrating competency-based education in the nursing curriculum. https://www.nln.org/docs/default-source/default-document-library/vision-series_integrating-competency-based-education-in-the-nursing-curriculumd6eb0a1e-1f8b-4d60-bc4f-619f5e75b445.pdf?sfvrsn=b37e7538_3

Nodine, T. R. (2016). How did we get here? A brief history of competency-based higher education in the United States. *The Journal of Competency-Based Education, 1*(1), 5–11.

Unger, L., & Sloutsky, V. M. (2022). Ready to learn: Incidental exposure fosters category learning. *Psychological Science, 33*(6), 999–1019. https://doi.org/10.1177/09567976211061470

Weinstein, Y., Madan, C. R., & Sumeracki, M. A. (2018). Teaching the science of learning. *Cognitive Research: Principles and Implications, 3*(2), 1–17. https://doi.org/10.1186/s41235-017-0087-y

3

Promoting High-Quality E-Learning Design and Delivery

Matthew Byrne, PhD, RN, CNE

Asynchronous distance and correspondence courses have allowed for learning at a distance with progressively more sophisticated media starting with mailed materials, radio and television delivery, on through cassette and VHS tapes until arriving at the early days of the internet with roots going back to the 1800s. The more rapid rise in the number of students taking online courses, starting early in the 2000s, was accompanied by an increase in online learning quality improvement research, online delivery standards, and organizations providing professional development services. Online learning beyond just single course translation was exponentially scaled in 2011 with the first massive, open, online course on artificial intelligence despite the term being coined three years earlier.

BACKGROUND

It would be impossible to talk about online learning without consideration of the impacts that the COVID-19 pandemic had for almost every teacher and student on the planet. During the pandemic, online learning became one of the safest means of providing instruction during the time frame in which vaccines were unavailable and the public health crisis was near its peak. Although there had already been large-scale shifts to fully online and hybrid delivery of courses prior to the pandemic, an editorial from the National Council for Online Education (2022) reported that 97 percent of US institutions had faculty members assigned to online teaching when they had no prior experience or preparation to teach in this way. The rapid transition to emergency remote instruction demonstrated that skill and readiness for online teaching and learning could not be assumed, required specific readiness steps, and could be enhanced by quality cycle processes and standardization (Altman et al., 2020; Zimmerman et al., 2020). A review of the online quality movement and best practices for high-quality online learning design and delivery can help faculty further improve their current and future e-learning practices.

Translating traditional face-to-face nursing courses to online and hybrid formats was fraught with issues even before the pandemic, which were often due to faculty skepticism, expansion of student workload, a lack of substantive interaction, challenges with engaging students, and negative impacts to student retention (Regmi & Jones, 2020; Wallace et al., 2021; Wilson et al., 2021). These issues, along with inconsistent evidence related to the educational efficacy and effectiveness of strictly online learning, did not help the perception of online learning as a lower quality delivery option (Baum & McPherson, 2019; Regmi & Jones, 2020). Postpandemic, the online quality movement continues to be part of addressing these gaps with a universal focus on improving the student learning experience. Online quality improvement efforts promote what Simunich et al. (2022) called a "culture of quality" in which continuous analysis and improvement become the faculty and institutional norm.

THE QUALITY IMPROVEMENT MOVEMENT

Baldwin et al. (2018) reviewed several types of online quality evaluation instruments and noted that "building a course without quality standards is like building a house without safety and building codes" (p. 55). The online learning quality movement was driven by concerns about the quality and effectiveness of online courses, along with faculty requests for resources and professional development to help them with the transitioning of courses. The two largest and earliest groups in this movement were the Sloan Consortium, which eventually rebranded as the Online Learning Consortium (OLC), and the Quality Matters (QM) group. These organizations and others like them offered a variety of fee-based services, including professional development, online resources, rubrics, and course review guidance, all of which focused on design of high-quality online courses.

Many universities responded to the growth in online learning by either buying into the proprietary quality resources and services or creating their own versions of them. The California State University Quality Learning and Teaching (QLT) framework and the University of Illinois Quality Online Course Initiative rubric are examples of homegrown models intended to address the quality themes shared by most pay-for-service models. All these tools vary in terms of the level of research that supports them, the type of rating systems they use for evaluation (e.g., some are just checklists), the quantity and type of criteria, and the domains covered within their criteria (e.g., design vs. delivery). The differentiation of design versus delivery is important because of the different considerations that go into each. Course design focuses on ensuring a fit between the key course elements such as outcomes, learning activities, and assessment/evaluation framework; delivery, however, relates to the implementation of the plan through teaching techniques, communication patterns, learning activities, and student feedback.

Online course development and e-learning resources have also expanded greatly since the 2000s through organizations such as EDUCAUSE and MERLOT as well as sites such as the Vanderbilt University Center for Teaching. Even learning and course management system companies produced resources, such as the Canvas Course Evaluation Checklist v2.0 (Instructure, 2019). The CCEC is notable in that it is aligned with several universal design for learning (UDL) principles (Baldwin & Ching, 2019). UDL principles are particularly salient in this context given that they provide evidence-based guidance for optimizing teaching and learning in any delivery modality, including online learning (Center for Applied Special Technology [CAST], 2018) (Table 3.1). More information about UDL is provided in Chapter 6.

TABLE 3.1

Universal Design Principles Applied to E-Learning

Principle	Application to eLearning
Course Overview	➤ How to get started in a course ➤ Introductions (faculty and students) ➤ Key documents and resources (e.g., syllabus) ➤ Overview of how the course is organized and delivered ➤ Policies and expectations are outlined, including communication and academic integrity ➤ Tips for being successful in the course are provided, including academic support services and institutional resources (e.g., advising, writing help)
Course Technology	➤ Technology requirements and tools to be used are outlined ➤ Listing of support services/help desk resources ➤ Skills and technical competencies for course and technology are presented ➤ Mobile accessibility and readability (if applicable) ➤ Privacy and copyright rules are published and followed
Curricular Design	➤ Course objectives, outcomes, and/or competencies are defined and measurable ➤ Learning activities align course objectives, outcomes, and/or competencies ➤ Universal design for learning principles are considered and followed in the design and delivery of course ➤ Supporting course materials are contemporary, relevant, and varied
Course Visual Design	➤ Consistent layouts that adhere to visual design best practices, such as consistent font types and sizes; sufficient contrasts of font to background; and use of white space ➤ Course navigation is evident ➤ Tables and slides are formatted for understanding and simplicity ➤ Media choices, such as images and videos, are inclusive and diverse ➤ Formats and design support a range of student abilities and needs and assistive technologies (e.g., captions and screen-reader friendly design) ➤ General usability principles are followed in course visual design and flow
Assessment and Evaluation	➤ Grading policies, including late submissions ➤ Rubrics and criteria for assignments provided ➤ Frequent, appropriate, and varied methods for students to ascertain progress ➤ Opportunities for learner feedback to faculty and about course ➤ Assessments align to course outcomes, objectives, and/or competencies ➤ Timely feedback is provided on assignments and via gradebook ➤ Examples of previous student work or sample assignments are presented if appropriate

(continued)

TABLE 3.1

Universal Design Principles Applied to E-Learning *(Continued)*

Principle	Application to eLearning
Learning Activities and Interaction	➤ Varied and with active, problem-based approaches that include real-world assignments ➤ Help students progress toward achievement of course outcomes, objectives, and/or competencies ➤ Supportive of collaborative work ➤ Student-to-student and faculty-to-student interactions promote community and trust ➤ Substantive interaction time is based on course length and type
Course Delivery (from Quality Learning and Teaching only)	➤ Identifies saliency within course content and learning activities ➤ Facilitates discussions, including disagreements and keeping students focused ➤ Faculty uses teaching techniques that promote student engagement, motivation, and new approaches to thinking ➤ Regular communication about the course and upcoming due dates and content ➤ Students are given opportunity for course closure and reflection

Thematically, the rubrics from quality organizations, university-created frameworks, and those published during and after the rise of online learning share many characteristics (Baldwin et al., 2018). Following is a summation of some themes found in the OLC Quality Scorecard v4.0, QM rubric (2018), QLT, and CCEC v2.0, all of which reflect best practices for creating a more standardized and high-quality online learning experience.

Critiques and Areas for Growth in the Quality Improvement Movement

The quality improvement movement is not without its critics. In looking at the rubrics, they can be lengthy. For example, the 2018 QM standards have 42 checklist items and the OSCQR 4.0 has 50 standards (Hollis, 2018; OLC, 2021). Translating previous courses or designing new courses for high-quality online learning experiences can be difficult even without having to also adhere to lengthy checklists and rubrics. Just as there has been criticisms of rubrics and their impacts on student learning and faculty practice, the quality improvement movement has also prompted concerns about a lack of opportunity for faculty innovation and creativity. The QM guide, as an example, notes that the rubric is intended to guide design of a course but not delivery. This leaves room for faculty personalization but may also be seen as incomplete guidance. Burtiss and Stommel (2021) posited that standardized and overly prescriptive approaches may further dehumanize teaching through adversarial relationships between administration, students, and faculty. Having strong online learning champions, working toward faculty buy-in versus mandates, and creating culture shifts toward quality can counter adversarial relationships and disengagement (Gregory et al., 2020; Simunich et al., 2022).

Evidence supporting the impact of quality work and standardization has shown mixed results (Esfijani, 2018; Regmi & Jones, 2020). For example, Gaston and Lynch (2019) found only trends toward greater student engagement in nursing courses that were designed using the QM rubrics. Historically, educational research can be very difficult given the large number of variables influencing educational delivery and outcomes. It is also important to note that innovations in teaching are difficult to create or prove improvements to student achievement. Evidence supporting quality work may similarly suffer from the challenges of proving or creating value with educational innovations (Barshay, 2018).

Creating high-quality courses is in some cases celebrated through achievement of certification or other similar designations. These efforts can improve standardization and quality but can also come at a great time and resource cost to faculty, especially given reports of a lack of insufficient faculty support and resources (Gregory et al., 2020; Regmi & Jones, 2020). For example, Bryan et al. (2021) described their largely positive multiyear efforts in a nursing program to improve online learning quality, including their process of becoming a QM member and working to achieve QM certification. The authors noted, though, that achieving and maintaining certification could be time consuming and frustrating in a constantly changing and accreditation heavy curricular environment like those in nursing programs.

One remaining frontier of success in online learning quality relates to equity. Online learning has been sometimes promised as an equalizing delivery modality that could better serve students with disabilities, racialized students, students experiencing poverty, and first-generation college students. Unfortunately, these populations are more likely to be disenfranchised and have disproportional outcomes with online learning (Baum & McPherson, 2019; Sublett, 2020). Organizations such as Every Learner Everywhere are a resource for advancing equity in online learning as well as CAST (2018), which created the UDL framework.

ONLINE LEARNING DELIVERY: BEYOND JUST DESIGN

The main quality improvement checklists and standards primarily or even exclusively focus on course design. Course design has a massive impact on the actual course delivery and faculty practice when it comes to student interaction, feedback, and facilitation of learning activities. Faculty may continue to need guidance and support, though, in terms of continuously evolving best practices for delivery of online learning and doing so in progressively more inclusive and accessible ways (Baum & McPherson, 2019; Sublett, 2020; Wilson et al., 2021).

Learning theories that are more delivery focused may also assist nursing faculty with online learning delivery (Picciano, 2017; Rembish et al., 2022). The community of inquiry (COI) model (Dawson et al., 2022; Garrison et al., 1999) focuses on social interaction and active learning. Because of the nature of nursing practice, it is a logical fit for nursing education (Smadi et al., 2021) given the mix of psychomotor, cognitive, and affective aspects of practice. The COI model proposes interaction and community as crucial to humanizing online learning. Faculty effectiveness must span the triad of cognitive, social, and teaching presence through careful selection and delivery of teaching strategies. For example, in an online environment, a faculty's presence is made known through timely feedback, discussion forums, collaborative creation spaces, advising, and course meetings through videoconferencing.

Harasim's (2012) online collaborative learning theory similarly centers on the interaction and collaboration aspects of learning, notably how it can be used for knowledge building. Learners use a variety of tools to collaboratively generate ideas, organize those ideas, and then reach a point of intellectual convergence that addresses the problem at hand (often in the form of an assignment). The readily available and low-/no-cost options for online collaboration have expanded for both informal and formal learning as well as for professional knowledge sharing across a variety of applications and contexts, as seen with information sharing during the COVID-19 pandemic.

The 6P4C conceptual model (Byrne, 2023) can help guide educators through design and delivery with an emphasis on humanizing the experience through the deliberate fostering of civility, communication, collaboration, and community building (the four Cs). These connective principles interweave the six key design and delivery considerations of the model (the six Ps), which include participants (learners), platforms available for delivery, a well-developed teaching plan, safe space creation for intellectual play, engaging and inclusive presentations, and regular progress checks toward learning. The 6P4C conceptual model uses rules of thumb and best practices in the form of design and delivery questions that can help faculty at the beginning, middle, and end of learning experience development.

EMERGING MODALITIES AND OPPORTUNITIES

The application of standards and best practices for online learning will continue to be an important part of ensuring high-impact and high-quality learning experiences. The application and revision of these standards in response to emerging modalities will be crucial in the continuing evolution of higher education. Delivery modalities that are more self-paced or that resemble hyflex (student choice of synchronous, asynchronous, online, or face-to-face hybrid learning) are not well represented in standards or in design and delivery models. Similarly, for nursing programs in particular, the integration of virtual simulation, academic electronic health records, and more competency-centered approaches continues to be on the frontier for research and best practices that will shape standards of online educational practice.

CASE STUDY

Bruce teaches a nursing informatics course that was converted to a fully online course a few years ago as part of the university's emergency remote instruction plan. He has been asked to keep the course 75 percent hybrid as a result of student feedback. Bruce completed a QM webinar provided through the university to edit the design of the course to be a more coordinated hybrid model. He applied the QM rubric throughout the refinement of this course and then met with a university instructional designer, who provided a critique of the course delivery components. The instructional designer identified that Bruce's course was suffering from "course and a half syndrome" because of the addition of even more content and readings when it was emergently converted to online delivery.

The instructional designer helped Bruce identify strategies to maximize the use of face-to-face class sessions through careful creation of online learning activities, technology, and collaborative work before and after the face-to-face sessions. Bruce was able to reduce content while keeping high-quality substantive interaction time and moving to a smaller set of high-impact learning activities. He was successful in getting the course QM certified and was pleased to see an increase in positive ratings across his student course evaluations.

CONCLUSION

The shift toward online and hybrid teaching has required educators to think differently about design, delivery, and evaluation of these learning experiences. Several quality improvement initiatives and guidelines have informed this shift with an emphasis on both fundamentals of teaching and quality components of teaching with more technology. The quality improvement movement for online learning has produced several rubrics and evaluation frameworks that can be used in conjunction with relevant theories and models to promote progressively more student-centered and impactful learning.

References

Altman, B., Shattuck, K., Simunich, B., & Burch, B. (2020). Quality assurance implementation: How it works. *Online Journal of Distance Learning Administration*, 23(4). https://www.westga.edu/~distance/ojdla/winter234/index.php

Baldwin, S., & Ching, Y. H. (2019). Online course design: A review of the canvas course evaluation checklist. *International Review of Research in Open and Distributed Learning*, 20(3), 268–282.

Baldwin, S., Ching, Y. H., & Hsu, Y. C. (2018). Online course design in higher education: A review of national and statewide evaluation instruments. *TechTrends*, 62(1), 46–57. https://doi.org/10.1007/s11528-017-0215-z

Barshay, J. (2018). The "dirty secret" about educational innovation. *The Hechinger Report*. https://hechingerreport.org/the-dirty-secret-about-educational-innovation

Baum, S., & McPherson, M. (2019). The human factor: The promise & limits of online education. *Daedalus*, 148(4), 235–254. https://doi.org/10.1162/daed_a_01769

Bryan, C. S., Oberlander, J. F., Reuille, K. M., Lewandowski, K. A., Topp, R., Grothaus, L., & Suh, S. M. (2021). Attaining quality matters certification for a registered nurse; bachelor of science in nursing program. *Computers, Informatics, Nursing*, 39(9), 484–491. https://doi.org/10.1097/CIN.0000000000000711

Burtiss, M., & Stommel, J. (2021). The cult of quality matters. *Hybrid Pedagogy*. https://hybridpedagogy.org/the-cult-of-quality-matters

Byrne, M. (2023). The 6P4C model: An instructional design conceptual model for delivery of e-learning. *Journal of Professional Nursing*, 45, 1–7. https://doi.org/10.1016/j.profnurs.2022.11.006

Center for Applied Special Technology (CAST). (2018). *Universal design for learning: The UDL guidelines*. https://udlguidelines.cast.org

Dawson, B. A., Kilgore, W., & Rawcliffe, R. (2022). Strategies for creating inclusive learning environments through a social justice lens. *Journal of Educational Research and Practice*, 12, 3–27. https://doi.org/10.5590/JERAP.2022.12.0.02

Esfijani, A. (2018). Measuring quality in online education: A meta-synthesis. *American Journal of Distance Education*, 32(1), 57–73. https://doi.org/10.1080/08923647.2018.1417658

Garrison, D. R., Anderson, T., & Archer, W. (1999). Critical inquiry in a text-based environment: Computer conferencing in higher education. *The Internet and Higher Education, 2*(2), 87–105. https://doi.org/10.1016/S1096-7516(00)00016-6

Gaston, T., & Lynch, S. (2019). Does using a course design framework better engage our online nursing students? *Teaching & Learning in Nursing, 14*(1), 69–71. https://doi.org/10.1016/j.teln.2018.11.001

Gregory, R. L., Rockinson-Szapkiw, A. J., & Cook, V. S. (2020). Community college faculty perceptions of the quality matters rubric. *Online Learning, 24*(2), 128–141. https://doi.org/10.24059/olj.v24i2.2052

Harasim, L. (2012). *Learning theory and online technologies* (1st ed.). Routledge. https://doi.org/10.4324/9780203846933

Hollis, E. (2018). Make a list and check it twice for quality course design. *Quality Matters.* https://www.qualitymatters.org/qa-resources/resource-center/articles-resources/checklist-for-course-design

Instructure. (2019). Course Evaluation Checklist v2.0. https://community.canvaslms.com/t5/Canvas-Instructional-Designer/Course-Evaluation-Checklist-v2-0/ba-p/280349

National Council for Online Education. (2022). Emergency remote instruction is not quality online learning. https://www.insidehighered.com/views/2022/02/03/remote-instruction-and-online-learning-arent-same-thing-opinion

Online Learning Consortium. (2021). Overview and information—OSCQR—SUNY online course quality review rubric. https://oscqr.suny.edu/evidence-examples/overview-and-information/

Picciano, A. (2017). Theories and frameworks for online education: Seeking an integrated model. *Online Learning, 21*(3), 166–190. https://doi.org/10.24059/olj.v21i3.1225

Quality Matters. (2018). Quality matters higher education rubric. Retrieved from https://www.qualitymatters.org/sites/default/files/PDFs/StandardsfromtheQMHigherEducationRubric.pdf

Regmi, K., & Jones, L. (2020). A systematic review of the factors—enablers and barriers—affecting e-learning in health sciences education. *BMC Medical Education,* 20(1), 91. https://doi.org/10.1186/s12909-020-02007-6

Rembish, M., Snyder, M., Sarage, D., Spadafora, N., & Alexander, I. M. (2022). Transforming clinical education during a global pandemic: Building new approaches to clinical education. *Nursing Education Perspectives, 43*(5), 325–327. https://doi.org/10.1097/01.NEP.0000000000001018

Simunich, B., McMahon, E. A., Hopf, L., Altman, B. W., & Zimmerman, W. A. (2022). Creating a culture of online quality: The people, policies, and processes that facilitate institutional change for online course quality assurance. *American Journal of Distance Education, 36*(1), 36–52. https://doi.org/10.1080/08923647.2021.2010021

Smadi, O., Chamberlain, D., Shifaza, F., & Hamiduzzaman, M. (2021). A community of inquiry lens into nursing education: The educators' experiences and perspectives from three australian universities. *Nurse Education in Practice, 54,* 103114. https://doi.org/10.1016/j.nepr.2021.103114

Sublett, C. (2020). Distant equity: The promise and pitfalls of online learning for students of color in higher education. *American Council on Education.* https://www.equityinhighered.org/resources/ideas-and-insights/distant-equity-the-promise-and-pitfalls-of-online-learning-for-students-of-color-in-higher-education

Wallace, S., Schuler, M. S., Kaulback, M., Hunt, K., & Baker, M. (2021). Nursing student experiences of remote learning during the COVID-19 pandemic. *Nursing Forum, 56*(3), 612–618. https://doi.org/10.1111/nuf.12568

Wilson, J. L., Hensley, A., Culp-Roche, A., Hampton, D., Hardin-Fanning, F., & Thaxton-Wiggins, A. (2021). Transitioning to teaching online during the COVID-19 Pandemic. *SAGE Open Nursing, 7.* https://doi.org/10.1177/23779608211026137

Zimmerman, W., Altman, B., Simunich, B., Shattuck, K., & Burch, B. (2020). Evaluating online course quality: A study on implementation of course quality standards. *Online Learning, 24*(4), 147–163. https://doi.org/10.24059/olj.v24i4.2325

4

Infusing Technology in the Classroom: Consider the Verb

Jennifer O'Rourke, PhD, APRN, CHSE

Technology has and will continue to transform nursing education, and educators need to be competent in teaching with and about technology. As a leader in promoting excellence in nursing education, the National League for Nursing (NLN) has long called for the adoption of technology as a tool to reframe how we teach and engage in both the academic and practice side of nursing (Nursing Education Perspectives, 2015). In 2016 and again in 2021, Wolters Kluwer and the NLN conducted a survey of nursing faculty to assess technology adoption across nursing schools (Wolters Kluwer & National League for Nursing, 2021). Not surprisingly, 73 percent of programs reported going online during the COVID-19 pandemic, and 91 percent of respondents indicated they are using virtual simulation and plan to invest more to continue to grow simulation within their program. Other technology endorsed by the respondents postpandemic included eportfolios, mobile apps, video software, adaptive quizzing, electronic health records, and makerspaces (Fig. 4.1).

A connected classroom uses technology to connect concepts for students (Barkley & Howell Major, 2022). The key to a connected classroom is the interactivity and engagement that is created using technology. However, that can be a double-edged sword if the technology is not intentionally and strategically implemented. What makes for successful implementation? Successful implementation starts with well-constructed SMART (specific, measurable, achievable, relevant, time bound) learning objectives. Well-written objectives help faculty make clear what learning goals are expected to be achieved — in other words, the goals answer the question, "Why are we doing this activity?" This chapter will walk through how to align technology tools to learning objectives and cite examples of technology tools.

SMART OBJECTIVES

A learning objective is a descriptive statement of what learners will take away from the class. Well-written objectives assist faculty in designing the overall course and individual components of the course (such as weekly modules); at the most specific level, well-written objectives can be used to align course activities to the content delivered.

Virtual, Secure, and Data Driven

Wolters Kluwer and the National League for Nursing (NLN) jointly conducted the Future of Technology in Nursing Education survey. The survey was undertaken in late 2020 to understand the shifts in technology adoption related specifically to the COVID-19 global pandemic through 2025.

Deans and faculty were surveyed to learn their plans for technology investment during the next 5 years and explore the barriers and opportunities related to those investments.

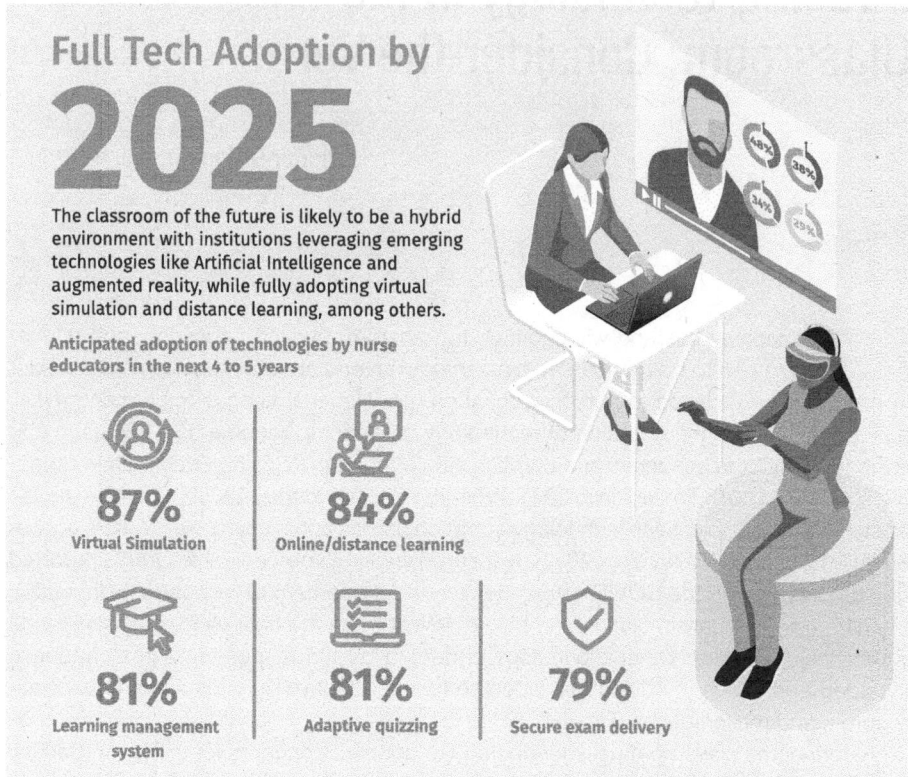

Full Tech Adoption by

2025

The classroom of the future is likely to be a hybrid environment with institutions leveraging emerging technologies like Artificial Intelligence and augmented reality, while fully adopting virtual simulation and distance learning, among others.

Anticipated adoption of technologies by nurse educators in the next 4 to 5 years

87%
Virtual Simulation

84%
Online/distance learning

81%
Learning management system

81%
Adaptive quizzing

79%
Secure exam delivery

FIGURE 4.1 The Classroom of the Future 2025. (Reprinted from Wolters Kluwer. [2021]. Forecast for the future: Technology trends in nursing education. https://www.wolterskluwer.com/en/solutions/lippincott-nursing-faculty/dean-survey; see the complete infographic at https://assets.contenthub.wolterskluwer.com/api/public/content/fb23da30a1eb44ab9155fca6cdac046e)

Module or individual weekly objectives should be aligned to the course objectives and ultimately the program goals or outcomes. In contrast to learning objectives, which are specific statements, program goals and outcomes are more general statements about what learners will gain from the course.

As the title of this chapter suggests, when integrating technology into the class, consider the verb when creating effective student learning objectives. Bloom taxonomy is likely familiar, and instructors use it often in developing and implementing their courses. The original Bloom taxonomy was developed in 1956 and consisted of six categories: knowledge, comprehension, application, analysis, synthesis, and evaluation (Bloom & Krathwohl, 1956). The taxonomy was later revised to reflect outcome-based objectives that are written using active verbs and with new categories: remember, understand, apply, analyze, evaluate, and create (Anderson & Krathwohl, 2001).

As you design your learning objectives, consider the verb and if your objective is SMART. Because writing SMART objectives is not always intuitive, especially for novice faculty, one recommendation is to utilize tools to help generate them. SMART templates are easily accessible on the web, but with the advent of artificial intelligence, writing clear objectives has gotten even easier. For example, when writing this chapter (think Fall 2023 for context), ChatGPT was used to write a SMART objective on "nursing students performing hand hygiene" (ChatGPT, n.d.). In less than three seconds the following was displayed:

Specific: Master and consistently apply proper hand hygiene techniques.

Measurable: Demonstrate a 100 percent proficiency in the step-by-step execution of hand hygiene protocols during random assessments and practical evaluations.

Achievable: Engage in regular hand hygiene training sessions, actively participate in hands-on practice, seek feedback, and utilize available resources, such as visual aids and instructional materials.

Relevant: Prioritize personal and patient safety by cultivating a habit of effective hand hygiene, contributing to a healthier learning environment and improved infection prevention.

Time Bound: Attain 100 percent proficiency in hand hygiene techniques within the next two months, with ongoing self-assessment and peer feedback incorporated into the learning process.

Example: "Through active participation in training sessions, consistent hands-on practice, and utilization of available resources, demonstrate 100 percent proficiency in the proper execution of hand hygiene techniques within the next two months, as assessed through random evaluations and practical assessments."

Does this match what you would have drafted? The example objective may seem a bit more complex than what you might draft for a class lesson; however, it does provide a great place to begin. This is also a great example of how emerging technology can inform our practice as educators in a positive way.

A WORD ON MAPPING

As discussed in Chapter 2, an effective strategy is to begin with the end in mind — that is, use the learning objectives as the starting point to identify the most effective teaching strategies and technology to promote competency development. A curriculum map is an effective tool to capture this process on a larger scale. When faculty think of curriculum mapping, they may think broadly with an eye on accreditation, overall program evaluation, and in 2022–2025 a major focus on mapping student learning objectives to the American Association of Colleges of Nursing (2021) *Essentials*. Although this is paramount for the success of an accredited nursing program, mapping at the local (course) level is equally as important. This is often called creating a course blueprint or class lesson plan. Begin with the end in mind, and ask yourself, "What do I want my learners to get out of today's class?"

TABLE 4.1					
Sample Class Lesson Plan					
Preclass Preparatory Work for Students	**Timeline**	**Learning Objectives**	**Inclass Activities**	**Technology Tool**	**Evaluation**

Minimum components of a lesson plan include student learning objectives, class activities, and an evaluation plan (Moore-Cox, 2017). Additional components may include preparatory materials for students to complete ahead of the class, a timeline of the class activities, and (pertinent to this chapter) technology tools and steps to use in class (Table 4.1).

ALIGNING THE VERB WITH THE TECHNOLOGY TOOL

As a certified course reviewer for Quality Matters (QM), a US based organization that specializes in standards and process for quality assurance in the design of online and blended learning, this author focuses attention on areas that include alignment between course learning objectives and course activities. QM defines alignment as the way "critical elements work together to ensure learners achieve desired learning outcomes" (QM, 2023). An easy way to understand the concept of alignment is to look at examples where alignment is not clear. Read the learning objectives and matched activities in Table 4.2 and ask yourself, "Will this activity help the learner understand the class content?"

Hint: One of the activities listed in Table 4.2 does not align well with the objective. The verb "compare" falls under the revised Bloom taxonomy of evaluate. Here a learner would be expected to first understand acid-base balance and then compare three primary mechanisms. Although a quizzing tool such as iClicker could help the learner

TABLE 4.2	
Quiz Yourself on Objectives	
Module Objective	**Activity**
Compare the three main mechanisms that contribute to maintaining acid-base balance.	Quizzing tool such as Kahoot
Explain differences between respiratory alkalosis and respiratory acidosis.	Video tool such as Panopto
Select an appropriate intervention for a postoperative patient experiencing respiratory distress.	Virtual simulation

TABLE 4.3

Examples of Technology Tools

Example	Type of Technology	Website
ATI	Simulation	atitesting.com
Body Interact	Simulation	bodyinteract.com
Canva	Graphic design	canva.com
EdPuzzle	Video	edpuzzle.com
EHR Go	Electronic health care records	ehrgo.com
Flip	Video	info.flip.com
Gimkit	Gamification	gimkit.com
Google Forms	Survey	classroom.google.com
Hoonii	Escape room	hoonii.com
iClicker	Polling	https://www.iclicker.com/
Jotform	Quizzing	www.jotform.com
Kahoot	Quizzing	https://kahoot.it/
Lippincott DocuCare	Electronic health care records	https://www.wolterskluwer.com/
Mentimeter	Polling	mentimeter.com
Montgomery College	Simulation	montgomerycollege.edu
Nearpod	Gamification	nearpod.com
Oxford Medical	Simulation	oxfordmedicalsimulation.com
Padlet	Discussion board	https://padlet.com/
Peardeck	Interactive slides	peardeck.com
Quizlet	Flashcards	quizlet.com
Shadow Health	Simulation	https://evolve.elsevier.com/cs/
Socrative	Quizzing	socrative.com
Study Stack	Flashcards	studystack.com
Trello	Note taking	trello.com
Vevox	Polling	vevox.com
vSim for Nursing	Simulation	https://www.wolterskluwer.com/
Wordwall	Gamification	wordlwall.net

identify discrete components of acid-base balance, it is less useful in helping a learner put the pieces together to form a mental representation of the three mechanisms. A better activity might be to use breakout rooms and have small groups use Google Teams to draw out the three mechanisms and then share with the class.

In the second example in Table 4.2, the verb "explain" could be aligned with an activity where small groups of learners work in a breakout room to create a short Panopto video of what respiratory alkalosis and acidosis are and then present to the larger class. This type of activity, using video technology, would support explaining concepts and relationships. Virtual simulation is an excellent technology tool for case-based learning and well aligned with the objective of selecting an appropriate intervention common in nursing. Several other technology tools could also align to this example, such as a polling tool using case-based questions and even an escape room where learners could take a series of steps with clues to reach the step of selecting an intervention.

CONCLUSION

Later chapters of this book (Chapters 8 through 17) each describe a specific technology tool, identify its advantages and challenges, and map a learner objective to that tool and an evaluation method. Examples of additional types of technology are included in Table 4.3; these can be vetted by faculty when selecting the best tool for their course. Happy mapping!

References

American Association of Colleges of Nursing. (2021). The Essentials: Core competencies for professional nursing education. Accessible online at https://www.aacnnursing.org/Portals/0/PDFs/Publications/Essentials-2021.pdf

Anderson, L. W., & Krathwohl, D. R. (2001) *A taxonomy for learning, teaching, and assessing: A revision of Bloom's taxonomy of educational objectives*. Longman.

Barkley, E., & Howell Major, C. (2022). *Engaged teaching: A handbook for college faculty*. Jossey-Bass.

Bloom, B. S., & Krathwohl, D. R. (1956). *Taxonomy of educational objectives: The classification of educational goals, by a committee of college and university examiners. Handbook I: Cognitive domain*. Longmans, Green.

ChatGPT. (n.d.). https://openai.com/chatgpt

Moore-Cox, A. (2017). Lesson plans: Road maps for the active learning classroom. *The Journal of Nursing Education*, *56*(11), 697–700, https://doi.org/10.3928/01484834-20171020-12

Nursing Education Perspectives. (2015). NLN releases a vision for the changing faculty role: preparing students for the technological world of health care. *Nursing Education Perspectives*, *36*(2), 134.

Quality Matters. (2023). Quality matters. https://www.qualitymatters.org

Wolters Kluwer & National League for Nursing. (2021). *Forecast for the future: Technology trends in nursing education*. https://www.wolterskluwer.com/en/solutions/lippincott-nursing-faculty/dean-survey

5

Learning Environment and Experience: Engagement, Motivation, and Community Building

Andrew Bobal, EdD

Although technology is a phenomenal tool and there are many examples of successful implementation, we would be remiss as technology leaders if we did not address the intrinsic and extrinsic factors that influence its success or lack thereof. A learner's motivation to succeed and want to learn is a main variable that contributes to academic success and the overall learning environment. The push to motivate learners and focus on evidence-based teaching practices is nothing new to nursing education. These pedagogical sentiments were being echoed prepandemic. Mastrian et al. (2011) wrote that "nurse educators need to commit to the implementation of evidence-based teaching practices and commit to developing the science of nursing education" (p. 5). More recently, Sapri et al. (2022) found that educational interventions improved nurses' evidence-based practice knowledge, attitude, skills, confidence, and behavior. It is integral for educators to be mindful of practices and approaches to improve the learning experience for the modern student.

THE INTERSECTION OF MOTIVATION AND ENGAGEMENT

Factors that contribute to motivation can be classified as either intrinsic or extrinsic (Oliveira et al., 2022). Although you as the instructor/creator have some control over the extrinsic component, learners have external variables other than schoolwork and academic success. Ideally, this allows us to affect the intrinsic variable to a degree. Are your students motivated to succeed in the course/learning? What do you do to motivate them? You are the cheerleader of the instructional environment. Encourage your students to succeed and give it their best. This extrinsic push will light the fire of the intrinsic side. Also, intrinsic motivation can result from many factors. Learners likely have experiences in their life that motivated them to succeed within the profession, or some may have been forced into this learning space. Whose intrinsic motivation is going to be greater? This chapter examines strategies to foster intrinsic and extrinsic motivation inside your learning environment. We will also outline best practices for building engagement and community within these environments, which can foster motivation for learners.

One can argue that a motivated learner is an engaged learner. Lu et al. (2022) mentions the importance of engagement within a learning setting: "Student engagement, labelled the 'holy grail of learning,' has been deemed vital in the learning process and linked to positive learning outcomes" (p. 1667). Their work saw the interchangeability of engagement and involvement and spoke of being involved on campus, not just engagement in a course. This sense of involvement can breed community and engagement. This notion is nothing new and speaks to another contribution: Astin's (1984/1999) involvement theory:

> The principal advantage of the student involvement theory over traditional pedagogical approaches (including the subject-matter, the resource, and the individualized or eclectic theories) is that it directs attention away from subject matter and technique and toward the motivation and behavior of the student (p. 529).

Astin's notion echoes the theme of this chapter. We need to rise above the traditional approaches and direct attention to the motivation of students and their behaviors. If a student is motivated to do well in the course/learning environment, then the student will be engaged in class, asking questions, volunteering, participating in discussions, and committed. What else does an engaged learner look like? Of course, there is some overlap within face-to-face, online, and hybrid environments.

Let us try an exercise. Close your eyes and picture yourself in front of the classroom of learners. If you teach online, picture yourself looking at the gallery view of your chosen web platform. What are your engaged learners doing? What are they not doing? If we went back to our inner Bob Ross, what does that picture look like? In the classroom, students maintain eye contact, following you around the room (hopefully you are moving), the learners are nodding along with your teachings, and they are displaying active listening by raising their hands when questions are asked. In an online environment, some of these same nuances are true, but the camera is your gateway to observing these behaviors. I always encourage learners to turn on their camera. I compare it to a learner coming to your classroom, putting on sunglasses, and laying down their head. This ideally would not be allowed in that environment, so in a virtual environment the camera is a key component to observing engaged behaviors and being able to read the room. Set the expectations for that environment and your learner.

DEFINING ENGAGEMENT IN EDUCATIONAL THEORY AND RESEARCH

Kearsley and Shneiderman (1998) developed the engagement theory. This framework for technology-based learning and teaching has much in common with other theoretical educational frameworks. Constructivist approaches to situated learning theory and nature theories of adult learning frameworks all consist within this principle. Kearsley and Shneiderman (1998) explain:

> Students must be meaningfully engaged in learning activities through interaction with others and worthwhile tasks. ... [W]e believe that technology can facilitate engagement in ways

which are difficult to achieve otherwise. So, engagement theory is intended to be a conceptual framework for technology-based learning and teaching (p. 20).

Engaging your students can be performed in a variety of ways, but most importantly, it is meaningful. Kowitlawakul et al. (2022) stated that "ensuring student engagement and motivation for learning activities is essential when using Edtech" (p. 263). Barkley and Major (2020) defined engagement as "the mental state students are in while learning, representing the intersection of feeling and thinking" (p. 6). There needs to be planning involved to foster the engagement within settings. As an educator this is an internal dialogue conversation in the planning of the lesson. Of course, there are many approaches and educational theories that speak to this planning process and what instruction looks like. A pillar of that conversation begins within Gagné's (1985, 1992) nine events of instruction. These developed conditions of learning come full circle to grasp the importance of planning, actual instruction, and reflection afterwards. These nine events (Box 5.1) are systematic and simple to follow. As users become more comfortable with them, these nine events can be combined or rearranged.

Wong (2018) used Gagné's nine events of instruction in teaching the Goldmann Applanation Tonometry. This diagnostic test helps identify people at risk of glaucoma. This instructional method was chosen because, "it is essential to pay close attention to the procedural tasks to ensure patient safety as well as reduce the complications associated with this procedure" (p. 45). Wong (2018) concluded, "The Gagné's nine events of instruction cater to different learning styles and help to facilitate the learning process. It provides a structured approach to formulating a lesson plan that is applicable to many other practical skills" (pp. 49–50). Of course, this is just one theory of education, and there are many out there, but one can see the important components embedded within most of these approaches. Additionally, although this book focuses on great technology tools and their integration within your teaching, one would be doing a disservice to the reader to not outline good teaching practices and approaches that can accompany these technology tools.

BOX 5.1

Gagné's Nine Events of Instruction

- Gaining attention of the students
- Presenting the content
- Providing feedback
- Informing the learner of the objective
- Providing learning guidance
- Assessing the performance
- Stimulating recall of prior learning
- Eliciting the performance
- Enhancing retention and transfer

Source: Gagné, R. M. (1985). *The conditions of learning and theory of instruction* (4th ed.). New York, NY: Holt, Rinehart & Winston; Gagné, R. M., Briggs, L. J., & Wager, W. W. (1992). *Principles of instructional design* (4th ed.). Fort Worth, TX: Harcourt Brace Jovanovich College Publishers.

Specifically looking at nursing education, Miner et al. (2015) looked at the effect of Gagné's events of instruction on student performance and course evaluations. Within an undergraduate medical-surgical nursing course, all faculty were previously just lecturing. Then, the authors took continuing education on Gagné's events and incorporated the practices into their instruction. The authors used student evaluations and mean course grades to analyze the effect of the different approaches of instruction. Chi-square analysis showed that student evaluations improved significantly ($p < .001$). Final grades did not measure meaningful change; however, ranges trended up, and the lowest course grades increased 4 percent, from 66 to 70 percent. These findings suggest an overall positive effect to incorporating Gagné's events of instruction. Some of these slight changes (e.g., "gaining attention" and "assess performance" of the learner) can make a substantial difference. Within the study, faculty started the class with a short video or comic strip. Additionally, as detailed in Chapter 8, to assess performance, faculty used minimal point quizzes (which could be made in electronic forms) to consistently assess learning during the course. These events are purposeful and orchestrated by the instructor. Although some of these types of events can be meaningfully planned, some of the dialogue and discussion in the course can be more authentic but also just as imperative as in "providing learner guidance" and "providing feedback." More recently, Chen and Johannesmeyer (2021) found "the approach (Gagné's events of instruction) accommodates active learning lesson planning, promotes transparency of teaching and learning, and is generalizable and applicable toward the instruction of various physical assessment procedures within the health professions" (p. 407).

Chen and Johannesmeyer (2021) spoke of the value of intrapersonal communication in its relationship to Gagné's approach. The instructional approach is meant to "facilitate instructor metacognition and knowledge building of applied through pre hoc, ad hoc, and post hoc reflection (p. 407)." Regardless of the medium, the engagement of students begins with meaningful forethought. This type of self-communication is not new to the orb of education. Dunagan et al. (2022) spoke of the importance of intrapersonal skills and self-growth by stating that "a focus on intrapersonal skills leads to personal growth and self-improvement, enabling lifelong achievement" (p. 145).

Imagine your outlook and the way you might communicate with others when you are in a bad mood or frustrated. That inner speech can be the springboard to both positive and negative interactions outside that personal dialogue. This could also be a conversation with colleagues and bouncing ideas off their experiences. Chohan (2010) added that "reflecting on daily teaching experiences, whether individually or with colleagues, provides teachers with an avenue to improve their teaching" (p. 17). More recently, De Jong et al. (2022), in his work with teachers in secondary schools, spoke of the importance of the continuous cooperative dialogue and its effects on learning by saying that "without continuity in collaboration, with teachers being absent or not engaging in experimentation, critical dialogues about teaching and student learning seem to have less impact on TPL (teacher professional learning)" (p. 1183). Not only does cooperative and internal dialogue improve the learning of students, but it also furthers the impact on the educators learning.

We can surely say what engagement is not. It is not just reading from your 40 PowerPoint slides as the learners sit stone-faced in front of you. Is there room for didactic lectures? Sure, there is a place for that, but it needs to be part of the tool kit. There needs to be the "why": Why am I using this tool or teaching method? And "because" is not an acceptable answer. Think it through, explore what might be best, and always ask for feedback. Otherwise, how do you improve? Consider framing that process around universal design for learning (UDL; see Chapter 6), which looks closely at the why, what, and how of learning (Center for Applied Special Technology, 2018).

BUILDING AN EDUCATIONAL COMMUNITY

A sense of community in a learning environment is crucial to success for learners. Learners who feel like they are valued, trusted, and included will be engaged in their learning and motivated to succeed in their learning. How does one foster this sense of community in learning? As with most topics discussed in this text, the sense of community and steps to creating it differ in face-to-face, online, and hybrid environments. One may argue that you must work even more diligently and deliberately to build this feeling of community within a strictly online environment. This building can produce tremendous results for overall learning but also universal retention and learners' attitudes. Capone et al. (2017) said that "sense of community is considered a core construct, capable of orienting interventions aimed at rising well-being within communities" (p. 375).

So how does one build a sense of community? Addy et al. (2021) discussed the importance of knowing the class. The authors created a "Who's in Class" survey form for students to complete at the beginning of the semester in an effort to "help instructors learn more about their students at the beginning of the course to better foster inclusively early, create plans for inclusion, and implement inclusive teaching practices" (p. 1). Instructors tried multiple strategies in the course to foster inclusion, including:

> Meeting informally with students one on one and weekly with groups

> Incorporating more flexibility at assignment deadlines

> Providing alternative virtual spaces for students to ask questions

> Creating classroom guidelines for instruction

Within their findings, Addy et al. (2021) reported many participants appreciated their instructor using the tool; 80 percent of the 220 participants wished the form were used by their other instructors. These findings suggest that students are conscious of the decision making of their instructors in fostering this sense of community. As echoed throughout this text, the meaningful incorporation of these strategies and tools is essential to student success.

Berry (2019) found that a sense of community for online students was influenced by their interactions in class, in study groups, and at in-person social events. Within an online environment, a learner needs to be heard. Opportunities for dialogue and discussion with various participants can mimic a social setting. Allow learners to learn from each other. These instances breed a feeling of confidence and comfort in the learners and thus provide the foundation for a learning community. Within this community is also the interaction between faculty and students. Berry (2019) states, "In an online program, faculty engagement with students can support retention. If programs want to strengthen the experience for distance learners, they would do well to consider how to support faculty in engaging with students outside of the classroom" (p. 189). Multiple scopes on literature come back to the engagement between the instructor and students. In or out of class, this crucial component to fostering a sense of community within a learning environment cannot go unrecognized. Martin et al. (2019) also spoke about the importance of the community within the environment. Within this research, eight faculty members who received awards for their online teaching participated in interviews. A sense of belonging and community is something that is authentic and needs to be meaningfully created. All the participants mentioned interaction or community as a key element in designing learning activities. They gave examples of collaborative projects, discussion forums, or peer review activities as necessary for students to interact with each other and the course content in different ways (Martin et al., 2019, p. 39).

The meaningful creation of community must be addressed within the design phase of the course. This is an area where the field of instructional design is crucial. Outside the course's overall layout and look, there are many resources available that outline best practices for online teaching and provide guides for creation. There are also experts across most campuses and organizations, with varied titles (e.g., instructional designers, learning experience designers, learning designers, instructional technologists) but all equally helpful. The role of these professionals and best practices within the field itself can fill a book. For this text's sake, however, let us look at some of the best practices for online/hybrid learning that can create engagement, motivation, and community building. These are the types of building blocks that you can incorporate into your instruction and ask for assistance in achieving from the professionals discussed previously.

BEST PRACTICES FOR ONLINE/HYBRID LEARNING

Engagement, motivation, and community building may look different in various learning environments, but at the core of these ideas, no matter the environment, is good teaching. An instructor must be motivated and engaged in instruction. If your course/class is missing these aspects, start from the beginning. What do you look like when you are teaching? What does your online environment look like? Let us take some time to discuss what this looks like in an online/hybrid environment. Although discussed within this chapter, this topic itself comprises an entire book. Check out *Best Practices in Engaging Online Learners Through Active and Experiential Learning Strategies,* by Smith Budhai and Skipwith (2016). This publication dives deep into the incorporation of experiential learning and active approaches.

At the core of best practices is the overall look and feel of the online environment. Clutter can be stressful for both learners and the instructor. The learner does not know where to look, and the instructor keeps getting the same email over and over about locating something in the online course. Darby (2019) said that "commonly, online students become confused, frustrated, and disengaged simply because you or the campus LMS (learning management system) have made it too hard to find the content and activities." Be clear with your learners, and make sure labels and dates are accurate. Additionally, today's LMSs provide a variety of tools and attributes that can aid in engaging and motivating learners within an online/hybrid community. Some best practices are outlined and discussed in this chapter. These instructional design exercises allow for community building to take place in the online course in a meaningful way. Is this an exhaustive list? No! These are just a sample, and with our teaching and technology world continuing to change and evolve, this is not a comprehensive list, but it is a great start:

▸ Develop clear guidelines and expectations for your learner
▸ Provide an area for Q&A interaction among learners and faculty
▸ Utilize meaningful tools (Zoom, audience response systems, LMS integrations)
▸ Be flexible
▸ Provide consistent and meaningful feedback
▸ Be conscious of accessibility standards/concerns
▸ Allow users to prove their learning in multiple ways
▸ Chunk your information

Now that you have some of this information, how can you learn more? And keep on learning. Thankfully, there are several free resources available that can improve online/hybrid learning. A good place to start is with LinkedIn. Not only can you connect with experts from all over, but the videos, resources, and content available within the platform are quite impressive. On top of the free resources available there are many opportunities to join member cohorts or academies to better teaching practices. Find some of your favorite resources and experts out there in the world of the web and connect with them, and build your personal learning network (PLN). Ask questions. Be vulnerable. Learn! A study completed by Trust et al. (2016) looked at the effect of PLNs for teachers and found that these networks can be exceptionally beneficial for those in the education field:

> Various teachers in our study indicated that PLNs afforded access to additional resources and ideas, collaboration with new and diverse colleagues, re-consideration of the very meaning of their work and identities, and even the support needed to stay in the profession (pp. 28–29).

More recently, Kumar and Nanda (2022) reviewed several social media sites as learning tools (e.g., LinkedIn). They noted the experiences, expertise, and knowledge available on the sites. This type of resource allows for professionals to break down the walls and learn from anyone, anywhere, "Moreover, LinkedIn provides opportunities to network with professionals around the Globe and going beyond the geographical boundaries" (Kumar & Nanda, 2022, p. 14).

CONCLUSION

If we want to keep on improving and be described as lifelong learners, it is integral to continue to grow and improve. That is likely one of the reasons you are reading this book. The process does not stop here, however; putting these tools and strategies into meaningful practice within your profession is your professional responsibility, so do it for your learners! Challenge yourself to be better and to learn new things. Think about your own teaching and how some of these tools and concepts can be integrated into the remarkable things you are doing daily.

References

Addy, T. M., Mitchell, K. A., & Dube, D. (2021). A tool to advance inclusive teaching efforts: The "who's in class?" Form. *Journal of Microbiology & Biology Education*, 22(3), e00183-21.

Astin, A. W. (1984/1999). Student involvement: A developmental theory for higher education. *Journal of College Student Development*, 40(5), 518–529.

Barkley, E. F., & Major, C. H. (2020). *Student engagement techniques: A handbook for college faculty* (2nd ed.). Jossey-Bass.

Berry, S. (2019). Faculty Perspectives on Online Learning: The Instructor's Role in Creating Community. *Online Learning*, 23(4), 181–191.

Budhai, S. S., & Skipwith K. B. (2016). Best practices in engaging online learners through active and experiential learning strategies. New York: Routledge.

Capone, V., Donizzetti, A. R., & Petrillo, G. (2017). Classroom relationships, sense of community, perceptions of justice, and collective efficacy for students' social well-being. *Journal of Community Psychology*, 46(3), 374–382. https://doi.org/10.1002/jcop.21943

Center for Applied Special Technology. (2018). Universal design for learning guidelines version 2.2. http://udlguidelines.cast.org

Chen, J. J., & Johannesmeyer, H. J. (2021). Gagné's 9 events of instruction with active learning: teaching student pharmacists how to measure blood pressure. *Journal of Pharmacy Practice*, 34(3), 407–416. https://doi.org/10.1177/0897190019875610

Chohan, S. K. (2010). Whispering selves and reflective transformations in the internal dialogue of teachers and students. *Journal of Invitational Theory and Practice*, 16, 10–29. https://doi.org/10.26522/jitp.v16i.3782

Darby, F. (2019). *How to be a better online teacher*. The Chronicle of Higher Education, April 17.

De Jong, L., Meirink, J., & Admiraal, W. (2022). Teacher learning in the context of teacher collaboration: connecting teacher dialogue to teacher learning. *Research Papers in Education*, 37(6), 1165–1188. https://doi.org/10.1080/02671522.2021.1931950

Dunagan, A., McGrath, A. L., Catanzano, T., Robbins, J. B., & Bhargava, P. (2022). Key components of a robust faculty development program: An emphasis on contemporary programming events. *Current Problems in Diagnostic Radiology*, 51(2), 143–145. https://doi.org/10.1067/j.cpradiol.2021.01.001

Gagné, R. M. (1985). *The conditions of learning and theory of instruction* (4th ed.). Holt, Rinehart & Winston.

Gagné, R. M., Briggs, L. J., & Wager, W. W. (1992). *Principles of instructional design* (4th ed.). Harcourt Brace Jovanovich College Publishers.

Kearsley, G., & Shneiderman, B. (1998). Engagement theory: A framework for technology-based teaching and learning. *Educational Technology*, 38(5), 20–23. http://www.jstor.org/stable/44428478

Kowitlawakul, Y., Tan, J. J. M., Suebnukarn, S., Nguyen, H. D., Poo, D. C. C., Chai, J., Wang, W., & Devi, K. (2022). Utilizing educational technology in enhancing undergraduate nursing students' engagement and motivation: A scoping review. *Journal of Professional Nursing*, 42, 262–275. https://doi.org/10.1016/j.profnurs.2022.07.015

Kumar, V., & Nanda, P. (2022). Social media as a learning tool: A perspective on formal and informal learning. *International Journal of Educational Reform*, 33(2). https://doi.org/10.1177/10567879221094303.

Lu, G., Xie, K., & Liu, Q. (2022). What influences student situational engagement in smart classrooms: Perception of the learning environment and students' motivation. *British Journal of Educational Technology*, 53, 1665–1687. https://doi.org/10.1111/bjet.13204

Martin, F., Ritzhaupt, A., Kumar, S., & Budhrani, K. (2019). Award-winning faculty online teaching practices: Course design, assessment and evaluation, and facilitation. *The Internet and Higher Education, 42*, 34–43. https://doi.org/10.1016/j.iheduc.2019.04.001.

Mastrian, K., McGonigle, D., Mahan, W., & Bixler, B. (2011). *Integrating technology in nursing education: Tools for the knowledge era.* Jones & Bartlett Learning.

Miner, A., Mallow, J., Theeke, L., & Barnes, E. (2015). Using Gagne's 9 events of instruction to enhance student performance and course evaluations in undergraduate nursing course. *Nurse Educator, 40*(3), 152–154. https://doi.org/10.1097/NNE.0000000000000138

Oliveira, W., Hamari, J., Joaquim, S., Toda, A. M., Palomino, P. T., Vassileva, J., & Isotani, S. (2022). The effects of personalized gamification on students' flow experience, motivation, and enjoyment. *Smart Learning Environments, 9*(1), 16. https://doi.org/10.1186/s40561-022-00194-x

Sapri, N. D., Ng, Y. T., Wu, V. X., & Klainin-Yobas, P. (2022). Effectiveness of educational interventions on evidence-based practice for nurses in clinical settings: A systematic review and meta-analysis. *Nurse Education Today, 111*, 105295. https://doi.org/10.1016/j.nedt.2022.105295

Trust, T., Krutka, D. G., & Carpenter, J. P. (2016). "Together we are better": Professional learning networks for teachers. *Computers & Education, 102*, 15–34. https://doi.org/10.1016/j.compedu.2016.06.007

Wong, Y. L. (2018). Utilizing the principles of Gagne's nine events of instruction in the teaching of Goldmann Applanation Tonometry. *Advances in Medical Education and Practice, 9*, 45–51. https://doi.org10.2147/AMEP.S145498

6

Universal Design: Using Technology With Inclusion in Mind

Jennifer O'Rourke, PhD, APRN, CHSE

Universal design for learning (UDL) and accessibility are philosophies that focus on extending access and inclusion in the classroom and beyond (Center for Applied Special Technology [CAST], 2018). Universal design focuses on designing to make environments, services, and products available and usable to the largest number of people. Accessibility focuses on ensuring accommodations to address technical, design, physical, or cognitive barriers. Both philosophies are important to understand and implement, using best practices, to create an inclusive and equitable learning environment for nursing learners. This chapter will focus primarily on UDL but will incorporate examples to meet the accessibility needs of learners. Concepts and examples of how faculty can achieve this are shared in this chapter.

PRINCIPLES OF UNIVERSAL DESIGN

UDL stems from a larger universal design (UD) movement that was oriented toward architectural design thinking. The term was coined by Ronald Mace in 1987 (CAST, 2018). Mace challenged the idea that all things should be designed for the average user. He believed that models for accessible and usable environments went beyond meeting the needs of individuals with identifiable disabilities.

The UD framework includes seven principles (Box 6.1). Although these principles were originally designed around the concept of architecture, they have since been applied to other disciplines, including education. These principles seek to increase access and reduce barriers for learners so that they may engage equitably in the learning process. Rather than focus on the typical student learner as the receiver of information, UDL challenges us as nurse educators to create a classroom designed for all.

CAST, under the leadership of Harvard lecturer David Rose, designed a framework for UDL after observing that teachers often had little guidance on how to support learners who were performing poorly in school. Rose termed this "curriculum disability" because the standard learning environment was not useful to acknowledge differences among students (CAST, 2018). The UDL is a framework for creating environments that address

BOX 6.1

Seven Principles of Universal Design

➤ Equitable use
➤ Flexibility in use
➤ Simple and intuitive
➤ Perceptible information
➤ Tolerance for error
➤ Low physical effort
➤ Size and space for use

Source: National Disability Authority (n.d.). The 7 principles. https://universaldesign.ie/about-universal-design/the-7-principles.

the diverse needs of learners and promotes flexibility in the ways learners access and engage with course content and master learning objectives.

The defining principles of the UDL framework vary from the UD framework in that it is based on neuroscience principles focused on the why, what, and how of learning. There are three main principles of UDL: (1) multiple means of engagement, (2) multiple means of representation, and (3) multiple means of action and expression (CAST, 2018). The why of learning, or engagement, is centered around affective learning and focuses on providing learner choice and autonomy in learning, optimizing the value of work, fostering collaboration, and developing self-reflection. Representation is the what of learning, focused on recognition and perception. The emphasis here is on the display of information and offering multiple alternatives for visual and auditory learning, as well as using clarifying terms and language. The principle of action and expression, or the how of learning, are the strategic networks used to build expression, communication, and action.

EVIDENCE TO SUPPORT UNIVERSAL DESIGN FOR LEARNING

An estimated 26 percent of students in higher education have a disability or experience a form of limitation (Stinnette et al., 2022). The most common condition is attention-deficit/hyperactivity disorder, among other primary learning disabilities (Statistica, 2022). The number of new learners being admitted to nursing schools with those same limitations has increased. According to Levey (2021), assumptions underlying the application of UDL principles in higher education include a consideration of the diversity of our learners today and the use of inclusive pedagogy to meet learners where they are. The role of faculty is to teach effectively without lowering academic standards and designing instructional methods that meet the needs of all.

Integration of UDL may better support student performance. Much of the current evidence focuses on outcomes in students with disabilities. In a 2023 systematic review of the application of UDL among education programs, including higher education settings, the use of UDL was beneficial with a statistically significant difference for learners who represented a spectrum of diverse classroom learners (Almeqdad et al., 2023). Greater positive educational gains were achieved when the three principles of UDL (engagement, representation, action/expression) were emphasized in the learning process.

There is some evidence to suggest that when UDL principles are applied in higher education to learners who do not identify as having a disability, student beliefs about attention, memory, and multitasking change (Levicky-Townly et al., 2021). Specifically, learners report increased motivation to learn and pay attention when they are told what to look for and what to focus on. They develop greater awareness of their actions in the classroom and feel more empowered with managing information and ignoring distractions. Further, Dean et al. (2017) reported that learning improves with the use of UDL-inspired strategies (e.g., interactive books, audience response systems, other resources) that are available both inside and outside the classroom. Clear instructions, the opportunity for feedback, rubrics, and storytelling have also been cited as strategies learners want faculty to use to create a more accessible and equitable classroom (Wells, 2022).

The design and use of technology tools in education have been shown to promote equality for some learners and in some contexts; however, a true inclusive classroom evolves from using principles of best practice. Educators need to be confident and competent to use technology to address the diverse needs and preferences of learners.

PRINCIPLES OF ACCESSIBILITY

Quality Matters (QM) is a US-based organization that specializes in standards and process for quality assurance in the design of online and blended learning (QM, 2023). There are eight standards that support higher education courses in meeting the QM standard. The standard that is most relevant to this chapter discussion is the accessibility and usability standard. There are six substandards that provide guidance to faculty in creating a course that meets the needs of all learners. According to QM, meeting the standard of accessibility does not guarantee or imply that specific accessibility regulations of a state or country have been met; however, they are an excellent set of criteria to use as a starting point (see https://www.qualitymatters.org/sites/default/files/PDFs/Standards-fromtheQMHigherEducationRubric.pdf for the QM standards and substandards).

Although the QM standards speak to accessibility of a course, they can be broken down and applied to the integration of a particular technology tool. At the most basic level, a tool such as PowerPoint or Google Docs should follow UDL guidelines for text and images that are accessible to all learners. For example, images should include alt-text descriptions so learners with a visual impairment can access the same information as their classmates. Color, underlining, and bolding should be used for instructional reasons rather than to convey meaning. YouTube videos, podcasts, and other examples of audio tools should include closed captions, and transcripts should be made available. The technology tool itself should be accessible to all learners, and alternatives used only if that technology does not include modifications for learners with limitations.

Some of the more recent gamification tools that are being incorporated into nursing courses may be more of a challenge to determine if it meets accessibility principles and/or may be more difficult to adapt as they are external resources. However, more and more organizations are including accessibility statements on their websites and may list ways the tool can be modified for select learners' needs. For example, the online game Kahoot includes an inclusion and accessibility policy on its website. The iClicker student response system similarly includes an accessibility statement and resources for learners with accessibility limitations, including an iClicker that incorporates Braille. According to QM, course multimedia and technology tools should facilitate ease of use rather than create barriers.

EXAMPLES OF APPLYING UNIVERSAL DESIGN FOR LEARNING PRINCIPLES TO TECHNOLOGY INTEGRATION IN THE CLASSROOM

Applying technology into the classroom should include a consideration of UDL principles focused on foundations of teaching and learning principles. This starts by aligning the technology tool to the learning objectives for that course and content area. A great place to begin is by developing a lesson plan that incorporates a check and balance of UDL principles and follows an implementation rubric. Examples of these tools can be found from the University of Illinois Chicago (Stapleton-Corcoran, 2022).

Here are some key areas to consider when selecting a particular technology tool into the classroom using UDL principles:

➤ Choose accessible technologies that can be easily accessed by all learners, including those with disabilities, and ensure that the technology is compatible with assistive devices, such as screen readers or voice recognition.

➤ Incorporate gamification (Kahoot, Wordwall, Quizizz) to engage learners. Information about their accessibility for diverse learners can often be found on the company website, and they be modified to meet the needs of learners with specific limitations.

BOX 6.2

Teaching Strategies for Implementing Universal Design

Multiple Means of Engagement
➤ Promote an inclusive environment by utilizing accessibility principles.
➤ Utilize a variety of ways to deliver content (e.g., reading materials, video, podcasts).
➤ Create opportunities for engaged learning in the classroom through partner, small group, and large group activities.
➤ Integrate opportunities for self-reflection of meeting course objectives.
➤ Use tools to do real-time engagement (e.g., iClicker, emoji use, online quizzing).

Multiple Means of Representation
➤ Utilize content that is visually modified by learners to meet their needs (e.g., PowerPoint slides that they can enlarge, PDFs that can be read automatically, video with audio control sound).
➤ When using images, use alt tag descriptions.
➤ Provide closed captions and transcripts for audio content.

Multiple Means of Action and Expression
➤ Offer diverse ways to submit assignments (e.g., through written or audio).
➤ Provide checklists as a weekly reminder of assignments.
➤ Provide options for physically interacting with the technology through use of hand, voice, or keyboard.

➤ Utilize a variety of technology tools to present and assess understanding of content because this caters to diverse learning styles.

➤ Provide opportunities for learners to engage with the technology at their own pace, and allow for flexibility in accessing and reaccessing that tool per each learner's need.

➤ Create collaboration in the classroom by using technology tools that promote active engagement and communion among learners.

➤ Use active learning boards to share content with the learners such as whiteboards and electronic discussion boards, which can often be downloaded and audio transcribed.

➤ Encourage multiple types of communication and expression methods, such as emojis, audio text to screen, and images.

➤ Incorporate digital assessment into the course through examples such as interactive formative reflections, quizzing, and real-time feedback.

Box 6.2 includes examples of additional teaching strategies to meet the three principles of UDL design in the classroom.

CONCLUSION

The American Association of Colleges of Nursing and the National League for Nursing have called for educational transformation and reform in nursing that creates an inclusive and equitable learning environment for learners. UDL principles provide guidance to faculty in using technology to engage all learners with the why, what, and how of learning. By starting with the end in mind and anticipating multiple ways of learning, faculty can foster a culture of meeting learners where they are.

References

Almeqdad, Q., Alodat, A., Alquraan, M., Mohaidat, M., Al-Makhzoomy, A., & Al, A. (2023). The effectiveness of universal design for learning: A systematic review of the literature and meta-analysis. *Cogent Education*, 10(1). https://doi.org/10.2218191. 10.1080/2331186X.2023.2218191.

Center for Applied Special Technology. (2018). *Universal design for learning guidelines version 2.2.* http://udlguidelines.cast.org

Dean, T., Lee-Post, A., & Hapke, H. (2017). Universal design for learning in teaching large lecture classes. *Journal of Marketing Education*, 39(1). https://doi.org/10.1177/0273475316662104

Levey, S. (2021). Universal design for learning. *Journal of Education*, 203(2). https://doi.org/10.1177/00220574211031954

Levicky-Townly, C., Stork, M. G., Zhang, J., & Weatherford, E. (2021). Exploring the impact of universal design for learning supports in an online higher education course. *The Journal of Applied Instructional Design*, 10(1). https://doi.org/10.59668/223.3751

Quality Matters. (2023). Quality matters. https://www.qualitymatters.org/

Stapleton-Corcoran, E. (2022). Universal design for learning (UDL). University of Illinois Chicago: Center for the Advancement of Teaching Excellence. https://teaching.uic.edu/resources/teaching-guides/inclusive-equity-minded-teaching-practices/universal-design-for-learning-udl/

Statistica. (2022). Percentage of US college students that reported select disabilities or health conditions as of fall 2022. https://www.statista.com/statistics/827023/disabilities-among-us-college-students/

Stinnette, L., Silbert-Flagg, J., & D'Aoust, R. F. (2022). Nursing students with disabilities: a guide to providing accommodations. *Nursing Clinics of North America*, *57*(4), 671–683. https://doi.org/10.1016/j.cnur.2022.06.012

Wells, M. B. (2022). Student perspectives on the use of universal design for learning in virtual formats in higher education. *Smart Learning Environment*, *9*(1), 37. https://doi:10.1186/s40561-022-00218-6

7

Evaluation of Teaching and Learning Applications

Matthew Byrne, PhD, RN, CNE

Digital, e-learning, and technology applications have proliferated in the wake of the ongoing transition to hybrid and online learning since the early 2000s. Faculty are often experts in their domains of knowledge and may be excellent educators as well. Competence in teaching with technology, though, is a different skill set that may vary even wider based on the faculty's experience, education, and access to resources within their institution (Aguilar, 2020; Haleem et al., 2022; Karolcík et al., 2017). Beyond comfort with technology, the process of evaluating and implementing new applications can be challenging given institutional constraints such as finances, the learning context, delivery modality, technical or instructional design support, and the ever-changing nature of the application landscape. Evaluation rubrics and guides can be a helpful way to determine the value of both current and future teaching and learning applications.

TEACHING AND LEARNING APPLICATIONS DEFINED

According to Anstey and Watson (2018), e-learning applications are a "kind of digital technology, mediated through the use of an internet-connected device, that is designed to support student learning." The terms digital application and e-learning application are sometimes used interchangeably and are parent terms for a variety of applications that may be used in a classroom, simulation laboratory environments, or within online learning scenarios. The types and uses of digital teaching and learning applications vary greatly. Some may be useful for individual learning activities or may be used as actual learning platforms with multiple functions. Examples include classroom surveys and responses, concept and process mapping, presentations, student/peer evaluation, collaboration and group work, communication and interaction, electronic portfolios, and video production. Digital teaching and learning applications can add value to face-to-face or online learning experiences by promoting student engagement, collaboration, active and problem-based learning, higher-order thinking, and the addition of new pathways for reaching the learning outcomes (Aguilar, 2020; Cekic & Bakla, 2021).

FACULTY EVALUATION OF TEACHING AND LEARNING APPLICATIONS

The ever-changing nature of technology presents faculty with the need to find new applications to support their teaching, to integrate new technology required by their institution, or to evaluate existing applications. The timing of faculty evaluation of applications may also vary. Faculty may want to evaluate an application before, during, or after their course as part of their postcourse quality cycle review. No matter the timing or rationale, there are several key considerations that play a role in determining the fit to context, match to students, and faculty readiness.

Faculty who are considering adoption of a new technology need to evaluate their competence, readiness, and factors that influence technology acceptance. Lai's (2017) review of technology theories identified several overlapping and evolving models, such as the technology acceptance model and the theory of reasoned action. A faculty's motivation and intent along with their personal characteristics (e.g., age, gender, experience, voluntariness of use) intersect with the actual design and usability of the technology that is being evaluated. The models explain that faculty will be more likely to reject a technology that does not meet their perceptions of usefulness, ease of use, or a high-quality performance of the technology.

Beyond faculty readiness, acceptance, and planning, faculty are focused on ensuring that the technology is a fit to learning needs and characteristics of students. The level of students, their digital literacy, and access to hardware and software may all play a role in faculty decision-making (Haleem et al., 2022). In online and hybrid learning situations, faculty may want to consider how well applications promote digital community, interaction, motivation, and overall engagement with the course content. Certain applications may also create more inclusive learning environments for those with physical, cognitive, and social differences, including those who may not be aware that they have disabilities (Rybin Koob et al., 2022). For example, a faculty member may need to determine if a video recording application they want to use allows for closed captioning or if a web-based quizzing application is compatible with screen readers, as these functions can be valuable even for those students without disabilities or accessibility accommodations. Cost to the student is another practical factor given that higher education costs are already concerning, and proposing licensing and use of an expensive application may be met with resistance. There are many web-based and device-based applications that will allow educators or those with an education (.edu) email account to have free or limited functionality access that could promote evaluation. Ultimately, faculty want to ensure that any application used within a course promotes greater student learning and achievement of learning outcomes.

Applications have to work for educators themselves, particularly when they may have to quickly learn and implement the application. Bonnel et al. (2019) offer a set of priority factors for faculty to consider when evaluating new applications such as their readiness and motivation to learn, evidence of application effectiveness, time investment, their menu of application options, and the support available for both learning and integration. A study by Karolcík et al. (2017) explored features of applications that were important to faculty and found that ease of understanding and ease of use were the top two. These are both central facets of overall application usability. Usability is a design concept that also speaks to ease of learning how to use an application, and the efficiency and effectiveness in achieving the goals of using the technology in the first place. Usability is a central aspect of evaluation particularly because it is commonly where most of the frustrating flaws within applications are found. If faculty struggle to learn how to use the application and there are design flaws that create frustration, the application itself may become a barrier to learning.

Faculty also may want to consider the overall fit of the application to the learning context and delivery modality in terms of what functions an application offers. In evaluating the fit of an application for a learning experience, it is helpful if faculty have a sense of what their goals are related to seeking, to use an application in the first place. For example, a faculty in a hybrid pathophysiology course knows that there are several complex concepts that often require additional examples for students. They may want to utilize classroom response software to engage students and to gauge student understanding when they are meeting face to face. The faculty would ideally like to identify how individual students responded, allow for students to use their own mobile devices or computers to respond, and allow for multimedia to be part of the questions (e.g., text, images, video). Having a list of desired functionalities in advance will help narrow lists of potential application options.

EVALUATION RUBRICS AND GUIDES

A rubric or guide may be useful for examining a single application or to compare multiple options to determine the best fit. Faculty will need to find a rubric or guide that makes sense for their situation. Despite some variation, most of them have similar themes. If the use case is to compare two or more applications, it might be useful to select a rubric and exclude evaluation criteria that does not apply. For example, if the application is not intended for mobile use, that criteria within a rubric could be excluded. Sometimes the lack of functionality for a given application is indicative, though, of its limitations for the current or future teaching-learning context. Rubrics and guides can also help faculty identify new functions that they may not have considered but that still have positive impact on the learning experience they are creating or revising. The comparison of three contemporary rubrics in Table 7.1 gives a sense of the breadth of evaluation criteria as well as the comparability of criteria across rubrics. This information can be used to give faculty a sense of which of these evaluation guides/rubrics might fit the contexts for evaluation outlined earlier. Although some of these factors can also be applied to evaluating a learning platform or management system, these were designed primarily for stand-alone or smaller scale applications. Many of these guides/rubrics also reflect technical functioning and use for teaching, whereas depending on the sophistication and type of technology, a review of the vendor may also be helpful. For example, faculty may want to work with their information technology colleagues to evaluate vendor services provided for integration, implementation, and postdeployment support; frequency of software updates, and whether system enhancements could be submitted (see Table 7.1).

TABLE 7.1

Comparison of Three Contemporary Digital Application Evaluation Rubrics and Guides

The Rubric for E-Learning Application Evaluation (Anstey & Watson, 2018) has eight categories with multiple subcategories and a rating system of works well, minor concerns, or serious concerns	The CEELTES has four categories with multiple subcategories, each with unique scoring (Karolcík et al., 2015)	The Criteria for Evaluating Workforce EdTech Applications (EdTech Center, 2023) has nine categories with a five-level scale related to evidence of meeting the criteria
Functionality (4)	Category 1: Technical and technological attributes (7)	Ease of use and navigation
Accessibility (4)	Category 2: Content, operation, information structuring, processing (6)	Accessibility
Technical (3)	Category 1: Technical and technological attributes (7)	Technical aspects
Mobile design (3)	Category 1: Technical and technological attributes (7)	Technical aspects
Privacy, data protection, and rights (3)	Category 1: Technical and technological attributes (7)	Data security
Social presence (3)	Category 4: Psychological and pedagogical aspects (13)	Features and design
Teaching presence (3)	Category 4: Psychological and pedagogical aspects (13)	Assessment Content Standards
Cognitive presence (3)	Category 3: Information processing in terms of learning, recognition, and education needs (four subcategories) Category 4: Psychological and pedagogical aspects (13)	Impact Content Features and design

CHALLENGES IN EVALUATING TEACHING AND LEARNING APPLICATIONS

Using a rubric or a guide can promote a more standardized and objective approach to matching an application to faculty need, learning content, delivery modality, and the student population. Many rubrics lack psychometric and effectiveness testing. As a result, ratings on rubrics and guides may not always correlate with educational results (Karolcík et al., 2017). Some rubrics and guides may also be outdated when trying to use them for emerging or more disruptive innovations (e.g., artificial intelligence applications). Gaps and validity of rubrics and guides and the nature of applications themselves may require faculty to evaluate applications being used for teaching at certain interval(s) while the course is underway or as part of the end-of-course faculty evaluation. It may be much easier to evaluate the criteria found in guidelines and rubrics given that students and faculty will have had experience with the application itself. Faculty may want to consider not only their critique of the application but perhaps, more importantly, to seek student evaluations of it as well. For example, if students were required to use a video recording software for group presentations, it will be important for faculty to think about the ease of setting up the software, tracking students' completion of work, and direct student feedback on ease of use. Important to note, evaluation is a continual process that does not stop after first use evaluation, which is especially salient with technologies that continuously evolve.

CONCLUSION

Just as expertise in an area of content does not imply that a faculty has commensurate skills to teach about it, a faculty's ability to integrate and evaluate technology must also not be assumed. Evaluating digital teaching and learning applications requires faculty to think about their own readiness and skill as well as the broader teaching and learning context in which an application may be implemented. Despite their limitations, rubrics and guides can help faculty determine the quality of new or existing applications as well as help in comparing potential options they may be considering.

Within the technology tool chapters are case studies that provide examples of how a technology can be implemented into the classroom. Discussion of how these case studies are implemented and evaluated are an important part in understanding the full use of technology. Remember, you are not alone in this work. Reach out to your colleagues and instructional designers or establish a technology workgroup to address some common use challenges.

References

Aguilar, S. J. (2020). A research-based approach for evaluating resources for transitioning to teaching online. *Information and Learning Sciences, 121*(5–6), 301–310. https://doi.org/10.1108/ILS-04-2020-0072

Anstey, L., & Watson, G. (2018). A rubric for evaluating e-learning applications in higher education. *EDUCAUSE Review*. https://er.educause.edu/articles/2018/9/a-rubric-for-evaluating-e-learning-tools-in-higher-education

Bonnel, W., Smith, K., & Hober, C. (2019). *Teaching with technologies in nursing and the health professions* (2nd ed.). Springer Publishing Company.

Cekic, A., & Bakla, A. (2021). A review of digital formative assessment tools: Features and future directions. *International Online Journal of Education and Teaching, 8*(3), 1459–1485.

EdTech Center. (2023). *Criteria for evaluating workforce EdTech tools*. Workforce EdTech. https://workforceedtech.org/tool-evaluation-criteria/

Haleem, A., Javaid, M., Qadri, M. A., & Suman, R. (2022). Understanding the role of digital technologies in education: A review. *Sustainable Operations and Computers, 3*, 275–285. https://doi.org/10.1016/j.susoc.2022.05.004

Karolcík, S., Cipková, E., Hrusecký, R., & Veselský, M. (2015). The comprehensive evaluation of electronic learning applications and educational software (CEELTES). *Informatics in Education, 14*(2), 243–264.

Karolcík, Š., Čipková, E., Veselský, M., Hrubišková, H., & Matulčíková, M. (2017). Quality parameterization of educational resources from the perspective of a teacher. *British Journal of Educational Technology, 48*(2), 313–331. https://doi.org/10.1111/bjet.12358

Lai, P. C. (2017). The literature review of technology adoption models and theories for the novelty technology. *Journal of Information Systems and Technology Management, 14*(1), 21–38.

Rybin Koob, A., Ibacache Oliva, K. S., Williamson, M., Lamont-Manfre, M., Hugen, A., & Dickerson, A. (2022). Tech applications in pandemic-transformed information literacy instruction: Pushing for digital accessibility. *Information Technology & Libraries, 41*(4), 1–32. https://doi.org/10.6017/ital.v41i4.15383

8

Keeping It Simple: A Review of Old But Dependable Tools

Andrew Bobal, EdD

This chapter explores old but good tools—the productivity tools we use daily as educators. Although these tools have been around for some time, they may be new for novice faculty. The goal of this chapter is to identify new ways to use these older tools, which have been referred to as Web 2.0 tools. More recently, some of these tools have been referred to as EdTech, which describes the comingling of using the tools with sound pedagogical principles (Kowitlawakul et al., 2022). Web 2.0 is an umbrella term outlined by Mastrian et al. (2011). These 2.0 tools refer to an interactive environment with connectivity and social networking, where producing and sharing are key. The five distinct categories of Web 2.0 tools are social networking and communication, collaboration, social bookmarking, e-learning, and services (p. 183). Kowitlawakul et al. (2022) stated that this type of instruction—integration of technology with research-based pedagogical approach—"helps to stimulate problem-solving and decision-making skills" (p. 270).

Let us dive deeper into the world that is dripping with collaboration and productivity and look at the tools that most of us have at our everyday disposal. There is no need to find something new and make a whole new username and password. There will be plenty of opportunities for that in later chapters of this book, which explore other tools. Chances are you already have one of these accounts, and you can start enhancing your learners' experience by using some of the features of these tools.

DESCRIPTION OF THE TECHNOLOGY

Let us start by looking at two powerhouses that are of the suite type within your organization or university. Both Google Workspace and Microsoft 365 (formally Office 365) suite are widely adopted within the field. Similarly, both pillars of technology have similar features and uses that can aid in our productivity and instruction (Gralla, 2022). It is recommended that an institution have a standard platform for use. Durand (2022) said that "choosing to standardize collaboration on a common learning platform creates an equitable experience for all parties—students, faculty and staff." Before we get into specifics and the research behind their uses, it is important to note that we will not cover all these applications in detail or the pricing models; we leave that to the information technology (IT) professionals, such as chief information officers and directors.

TABLE 8.1

Sample Tools in Google and Microsoft

Function	Google Workspace	Microsoft 365
Word processing	Docs	Word
Presentations	Slides	PowerPoint
Spreadsheets	Sheets	Excel
Data gathering	Forms	Forms
Collaboration	Meet/Chat	Teams/OneNote
Time management	Calendar	Calendar
File storage/cloud based	Drive	OneDrive

Google Workspace

The Google Workspace suite is not new to you but might be something now being utilized in a professional position rather than personal. This is a platform or set of tools that many of us have used because of the common use of email addresses (@gmail.com). You may have used only some of the available tools in the arsenal. Additionally, depending on the plan your university has purchased from Google, some of these applications might have distinctive features or not be present at all in your suite. Al-Emran and Malik (2016) stated, "Google has come up with a variety of constructive services that help the industry and education to perform their work effectively" (p. 85).

Microsoft 365 Suite

Like Google Apps, Microsoft 365 (formally Office 365) is familiar. The Microsoft suite has been widely adopted in higher education and in the business/private sector. Word, PowerPoint, and other programs directly installed on your local machines may be in the Microsoft suite. With advances in technology, these tools and functionality work online, too. They can then be synchronized with your local version to make saving and updating content from any device or machine seamless.

You can use the information in Table 8.1 to identify the different tools within both Google and Microsoft 365. You will notice that each suite has a competitor and that some of the names used are quite similar, which makes it easy to identify and reference when talking to another user.

EVIDENCE-BASED ADVANTAGES AND CHALLENGES OF THE TECHNOLOGY

These two cloud-based technology tools have long been compared to each other. Whereas Microsoft Word was first introduced in 1983, it was not until 2006 that Google even announced Docs and Spreadsheets (Google, 2006). Both products have only grown in features and effectiveness since then. A comparison of these products was documented by Skendzic and Kovacic (2012), who spoke of the advantages and disadvantages: "The greatest advantage of cloud computing is usage when the service is needed. And the greatest disadvantages are availability and safety" (p. 1751). These are still true today. More recently, Alam and Saiyeda (2020) acknowledged the higher education realm we are living in, saying "the paradigms of education have now shifted from traditional teaching methods to smart campuses with state-of-the-art technology and devices" (p. 41).

Advantages

Outside of the amazing productivity that comes from both these suites of products, students and faculty can collaborate on projects and cooperative groupwork on presentations and papers. Both are a one-stop shop for productivity and creation, and the uses are endless. For example, students can work cooperatively on a presentation that will be used in class; faculty can collaborate with colleagues on publishing an article, where they can work on the same document at the same time in various locations. Additionally, with wide adoption across education and corporate settings, there is certainly not a lack of resources and how-to information on either of these products.

Both suites offer mostly online tools that are linked to some subscription, usually through the university account or another purchaser. However, many of us get by with the free version of the Google suite products, which comes with a free @gmail.com email address. Important to note here, though, the distinction between personal and work access (e.g., if your campus uses Microsoft suite and a student tries to submit an assignment from Google Docs). A faculty member might have trouble accessing the submission, or the submission might not be run through the university tools for plagiarism. This is more common than one would like to think, so it is important, as with anything, to outline expectations for users' submissions.

The Microsoft suite can work with online products but also uses applications on local machines. This is true for Google, too, but mainly on Chromebook and other Android-supported devices. Additionally, most of the widely used functions in the suite are available in an offline mode that the user can initiate.

Recently, Opara et al. (2021) looked closely at the advantages and disadvantages of using Google Docs for online interviews within a qualitative data collection. They found "that Google Docs can be considered a viable alternative to the traditional face-to-face and telephone interviews" (p. 15). Within their research they use the Google Doc tool to conduct their qualitative interviews, allowing the user to work synchronously with the interviewer to capture responses. They also highlighted the cost savings that can be associated with utilizing this tool and its transcription technology: "As Google Docs interviews are transcribed verbatim immediately while being conducted, there are significant cost and time savings with the added option of conducting multiple interviews simultaneously" (p. 14). Do not fear, although this article outlines the transcription use on Google Docs, this same feature is available in Word products.

Challenges

A disadvantage of these applications is the constraint of needing an internet connection. Unbelievably, as I sat down to write pieces of this chapter, Office 365 Online apps were down all morning, so that meant I could not access previous writings and work on this project. However, the Microsoft suite has a leg up on that corner of the market because you can use all the programs on your local machine without an internet connection if you have them downloaded.

As previously discussed as an advantage for being widely adopted products, that can also make it cumbersome to shift through all the resources. Some videos or tutorials might be showing an older version, and the toolbars may be a little different now. Although a general internet search can yield millions of results, oftentimes the product website is a suitable place to begin. The videos and guides are more than up to date and show the most accurate representation of that product at that time.

Additionally, although outlined as a strength for Google suite, Microsoft 365 institutions need licenses for users to access the tools and features. The purchase of said products can certainly limit the availability of them for stakeholders. Also, if these are new tools to an environment, there is a learning curve involved. Most of us are familiar with Word, PowerPoint, and Excel, but a tool growing in popularity is Teams. Teams as defined by Microsoft is a modern workplace in the office, at home, and on the go. Although there is a free version of this tool, the main productivity and professional users come with a paid account. A research study recently completed by Hope (2022) used Teams within a pharmaceutical learning environment. Hope et al. (2022) stated the importance of having users willing to learn by stating that "people's willingness to learn new approaches and enhance their digital capability" aided in a successful study. Duffy (2023) adamantly stated, "Microsoft Teams is orderly and hyper-compartmentalized, but frustrating to navigate." Just like most technology, there is learning that must take place to be successful with the tool or space. Rarely can we jump right in and be successful immediately; patience and training are key aspects of a technology leader.

SAMPLE CASE INTEGRATION

To understand how to incorporate various components of Google or Microsoft into our everyday teaching and professional actions, a couple of examples are provided here for faculty.

Forms or Sheets

In most instructional designer roles working within an academic nursing program there is always some innovative technology to try, but we must pause and look directly at what we already have access to. There is a technology tool called Forms in the Office 365 world and Sheets in Google life that are valuable for nurse educators to understand. The tool on both platforms is remarkably similar and allows users to create writable electronic forms/sheets. Within the world of education there is a plethora of uses. For example, student understanding of weekly class content could be evaluated using a simple end-of-class survey created through forms. Table 8.2 includes an example.

TABLE 8.2

Educational Map: Integrating Office Forms

Objective	Implementation	Evaluation
Identify factors related to fluid/electrolyte balance across the lifespan	Students are provided a QR code at the end of the class session to complete the form on their device.	Course faculty review response statistics following each class session. Have follow-up discussion to clarify muddy points for learners.

Some of the instances of utilizing this tool can provide the instructor with meaningful real-time feedback. That feedback can be anonymous or tied to a user. In most cases, students are more likely to provide meaningful feedback when there is anonymity. Lim (2017) discussed the benefit of students anonymously submitting their exit tickets, stating this process "further enhances student motivation to participate as they know their voices are heard" (p. 406). In this manner, the tool is used as an exit or entrance ticket to gauge students' understanding or prior knowledge.

Additionally, another skillful use is designing the Form/Sheet to mimic an assessment. This allows students to practice questions in real time and gives instructors an idea of their understanding. This electronic method of gauging students' understanding can be more effective than the standard "does that make sense to everybody?" and nobody in the class responds. A study by Martin et al. (2019) looked at award-winning faculty and their online teaching practices. Within the study, "six of the eight faculty used quizzes either weekly or during regular intervals during the course to assess whether students were reading, understanding, and learning course content" (p. 39). Additionally, these award-winning faculty referenced the need for student feedback, in that "participants described mid-semester and end-semester surveys, student evaluations that focused on both course design and facilitation." The way the tool is focused on here is more of the formative feedback from students than gathered using these tools. Questions centered around their learning and where gaps might exist. Also, gauging their interest and prior knowledge of topics can provide valuable informative teaching data as instructors.

Furthermore, Form use is widely used in questionnaires and reporting of participants in numerous studies. Recently, a study by Addy et al. (2021) used Forms to create "Who's in Class," a questionnaire given to students that was designed to increase instructor awareness of learners and increase inclusive teaching practices. Overall, both instructors and students reported benefits from the tool. Additionally, Yeh (2022) looked at nursing student satisfaction within a flipped classroom model. Learners responded to the anonymous questionnaires in Google Forms for aspects of this mixed research study. These examples outline a use to create a better learning environment for all; the possible benefits of these tools include more than assessment and productivity. As you make your way through the various tools and strategies outlined in this text, remember to link to learner feedback and the productivity that comes with Forms in gathering that data.

TABLE 8.3		
Educational Map: Integrating PowerPoint		
Objective	**Implementation**	**Evaluation**
Describe respiratory acidosis, respiratory alkalosis, metabolic acidosis, and metabolic alkalosis	In groups of three to five, students work cooperatively to utilize PowerPoint to complete a presentation of key concepts of their topic area.	Course faculty review submitted presentations using provided rubric that outlines best practices. Other students also provide peer feedback on presentations.

PowerPoint or Slides

One of the most heavily used technology tools within the education realm is PowerPoint or Slides. These are the presentation tools that faculty use to build content and lecture material. Although some features vary across the tools, best practices of the presentations are similar. Table 8.3 includes an example of using PowerPoint for a class group assignment.

Although plenty of great presentations exist, and there are professionals using this tool to expert level, other presentations lack basic understanding of best practices and fail to meet some of the most obvious accessibility standards. Day (2021) spoke of the need for consistent structure in presentations and how that can aid in learners retaining knowledge: "The number one expectation from students on effective learning is having a clear structure to presentations" (p. 37). The author takes it to the next level by also recommending referencing this structure or framework throughout the presentation/lecture to inform learners of the progress (Day, 2021). We can equate this progress check to a completion summary or status bar—like pausing a show to see how much is left. Outlining the learning content in the beginning and then continually referencing back to that progress throughout instruction provides tracking guidance for learners. Furthermore, to echo the importance of structure of the presentation and overall teaching, prior research has found that PowerPoint itself has no pedological effect; several other factors contribute to positive or negative outcomes in teaching and learning.

Cullen et al. (2018) and Williams et al. (2017) agreed that PowerPoint has no pedagogical effect in itself and that it can lead to positive or negative results depending on other factors that may have an impact (Chávez Herting et al., 2020).

Like many other tools and technologies that will be discussed in this text, these too are simply tools in the tool kit. Good teaching is the backbone to students' success. As instructors, we owe it to learners to use these tools meaningfully and with pedological purposes.

EVALUATION OF THE TECHNOLOGY

The evaluation of this technology can be discussed at various levels. At the organizational level, IT directors and various other technology stakeholders within an organization would be making a commitment to the suite or software being utilized. It is crucial within these conversations that the teaching aspects and uses within classrooms are just as important as the productive tools of email and calendar. Of course, this text is much more focused on the former, and it would be advantageous for a participant to come prepared with the engagement benefits of the applications and examples of instructional integration. Additionally, for a single user or a smaller enterprise, the process and uses may be completely different. Some specific tools (e.g., Sheets vs Excel, Slides vs PowerPoint) might differ drastically.

In contrast, an instructor would evaluate the tool for the instructional needs and efficiency in the course. Take, for example, the use of Forms. What benefits can be seen incorporating this tool into the classroom? How can we avoid frustration or feelings of uncertainty for our learners? One clear benefit in evaluating the technology is the time-saving aspects. Juraev (2022) comments, "This valuable time can be used to work with struggling students."

CONCLUSION

Overall, these old but good tools aid in our daily productivity, but their potential uses across educational purposes for our learners puts them in a league of their own. Thankfully, with most faculty and students already having experience with these tools in some scope, the learning curve is small. Moreover, best practices can be the core of the conversation. As opposed to starting something brand new, the familiarity of these tools is unmatched across the learning environment.

References

Addy, T. M., Mitchell, K. A., & Dube, D. (2021). A tool to advance inclusive teaching efforts: The "who's in class?" form. *Journal of Microbiology & Biology Education*, 22(3), e00183-21.

Alam, M. A., & Saiyeda, A. (2020). A cloud-based solution for smart education: An extended version. In *Role of ICT in higher education* (pp. 41–50). Apple Academic Press.

Al-Emran, M., & Malik, S. I. (2016). The impact of google apps at work: Higher educational perspective. *International Journal of Interactive Mobile Technologies*, 10(4), 85–88.

Chávez Herting, D., Cladellas Pros, R., & Castelló Tarrida, A. (2020). Patterns of PowerPoint use in higher education: a comparison between the natural, medical, and social sciences. *Innovative Higher Education*, 45, 65–80.

Cullen, A. E., Williams, J. L., & McCarley, N. G. (2018). Conscientiousness and learning via feedback to identify relevant information on PowerPoint slides. *North American Journal of Psychology*, 20, 425–444.

Day, S. (2021). Maximizing PowerPoint: Best practices for adult learning. Department of Justice. *Journal of Federal Law and Practice*, 69(4), 33–38.

Duffy, J. (2023). *Microsoft Teams review*. PC Mag. https://www.pcmag.com/reviews/microsoft-teams

Durand, M. (2022). The benefits of standardizing collaboration tools in Higher ed. EdTech. https://edtechmagazine.com/higher/article/2022/06/benefits-standardizing-collaboration-tools-higher-ed

Google. (2006). Google announces Google Docs & Spreadsheets—news from Google.

http://googlepress.blogspot.com/2006/10/google-announces-google-docs_11.html

Gralla, P. (2022). Google Workspace vs. Microsoft 365: What's the best office suite for business? *Computerworld*. https://www.computerworld.com/article/3515808/g-suite-vs-office-365-whats-the-best-office-suite-for-business.html

Hope, D. L., Grant, G. D., Rogers, G. D., & King, M. A. (2022). Virtualized gamified pharmacy simulation during COVID-19. *Pharmacy*, *10*(2), 41.

Juraev, M. M. (2022). Prospects for the development of professional training of students of professional educational institutions using electronic educational resources in the environment of digital transformation. *Academicia Globe: Inderscience Research*, *3*(10), 158–162.

Kowitlawakul, Y., Tan, J. J. M., Suebnukarn, S., Nguyen, H. D., Poo, D. C. C., Chai, J., Wang, W., & Devi, K. (2022). Utilizing educational technology in enhancing undergraduate nursing students' engagement and motivation: A scoping review. *Journal of Professional Nursing*, *42*, 262–275.

Lim, W. N. (2017). Improving student engagement in higher education through mobile-based interactive teaching model using socrative. In *2017 IEEE Global Engineering Education Conference (EDUCON)* (pp. 404–412). IEEE.

Martin, F., Ritzhaupt, A., Kumar, S., & Budhrani, K. (2019). Award-winning faculty online teaching practices: Course design, assessment and evaluation, and facilitation. *The Internet and Higher Education*, *42*, 34–43.

Mastrian, K., McGonigle, D., Mahan, W., & Bixler, B. (2011). *Integrating technology in nursing education: Tools for the knowledge era*. Jones & Bartlett Learning.

Opara, V., Spangsdorf, S., & Ryan, M. K. (2021). Reflecting on the use of Google Docs for online interviews: Innovation in qualitative data collection. *Qualitative Research*, *23*(3). https://doi.org/10.1177/14687941211045192

Skendzic, A., & Kovacic, B. (2012). Microsoft Office 365—cloud in business environment. In *2012 Proceedings of the 35th International Convention MIPRO* (pp. 1434–1439). IEEE.

Williams, J. L., McCarley, N. G., Sharpe, J. L., & Johnson, C. E. (2017). The ability to discern relevant from irrelevant information on PowerPoint slides: A key ingredient to the efficacy of performance feedback. *North American Journal of Psychology*, *19*, 219–236.

Yeh, Y. C. (2022). Student satisfaction with audio-visual flipped classroom learning: A mixed-methods study. *International Journal of Environmental Research and Public Health*, *19*(3), 1053.

9

Gamification

Rebecca G. Davis, EdD, RN, CNE, CNE-cl
Miranda Smith, EdD, AGACNP-BC

Nurse educators incorporate gaming and quizzing technologies into classroom learning, as evidenced by the 10-fold increase of literature in this area during the last five years, with many studies published since 2021 (Meşe & Meşe, 2022; van Gaalen et al., 2021). Gamification actively engages learners' understanding and retention of course content and functions as a delivery method to present licensure exam-style items for practice and discussion. For this chapter, gamification will be defined as learning that includes common gaming elements of interactivity, challenge, and feedback into nongame events (Malicki et al., 2020). The use of classroom gamification has become more widespread in recent years because of the evolving technological capabilities of personal devices, although simpler instructor-led gamification technologies have been in use much longer (Reed, 2020; van Gaalen et al., 2021). For example, templates for classroom versions of Jeopardy, Bingo, and other simulation game shows and board games have existed since educators began delivering content using computers and projectors (Khaldi et al., 2023; McEnroe-Petitte & Farris, 2020). Clickers have also been widely used in higher education to gamify learning by allowing students to vote on correct answers to multiple-choice questions (Shapiro et al., 2017). Today, however, extra student purchases are not needed. The majority of current gamification tools can be operated via cell phones or other personal devices.

Moreover, nursing education may also be gamified during clinical experiences, simulation, and during independent learning and study time (Suh et al., 2022). Although less common, these additional uses of gamification may strengthen the community of learning outside of traditional classroom time by increasing student engagement with one another and increasing learners' self-efficacy (Chen & Liang, 2022). Quizzing will be the primary focus of this chapter because of its ubiquity in nursing education, its inclusion of multiple gamification elements, and its transferability beyond the classroom to other learning environments (Reed, 2020; Tavares, 2022). As many educators are already familiar with gamification in classroom settings, this chapter's case examples will illustrate ways to move gamification in nursing education into simulation and small study groups. Sample cases at the end of this chapter will discuss how the popular quizzing technology Kahoot may be used to gamify simulation prebriefing and debriefing discussions, and how technologies that simulate television quiz shows may gamify collaborative learning, whether in the classroom or within student-led independent study groups.

DESCRIPTION OF THE TECHNOLOGY

Classroom group quizzing technologies that deliver practice questions through polling platforms have become widely used among nurse educators (McEnroe-Petitte & Farris, 2020; Reed, 2020). Several current popular examples are Kahoot, Quizziz, Quizlet Live, and Blooket. The free versions of these gaming technologies allow instructors to deliver multiple-choice or true/false questions to small groups of learners who compete on their personal electronic devices, earning points for both accuracy and speed in answering. Depending on the technology, students may compete individually, in teams, or both. The payment structure for low-cost paid versions of these technologies offers additions such as more variety in question types, allowance of a greater number of players per game, and the ability to create an unlimited number of games. Nurse educators may use these and other quizzing applications to deliver questions like those on nursing licensure exams. Competition elements, such as winner podiums, leaderboards, badges, and achievements of streaks, keep learners engaged (Sarker et al., 2021; Wingo et al., 2019).

Quiz show technologies are educational templates that simulate popular television-based game shows, making the rules for play and scoring familiar to many students. Like polling-based quizzing applications, these templates allow nurse educators to provide students with practice answering nursing exam-style questions. Instructors additionally may introduce the NextGen-style questions to students through many of these platforms. Students can work collaboratively in some of these platforms and receive immediate feedback on answers prior to seeing the NextGen-style questions on a standardized assessment. In classrooms, questions are frequently projected on a screen in the style of a popular game show. Teams of students may then compete against each other fostering clinical judgment through collaborative discussion and problem-solving (Zehler & Musallam, 2021). Educators may also prepare independent quizzing games for students to use as independent learning tools within study groups as an alternative to creating study guides or lists of content to study (García-Viola et al., 2019; Suh et al., 2022). In our college's prelicensure nursing programs, many of our teaching teams create and share these types of games with students as a study resource.

EVIDENCE-BASED ADVANTAGES AND CHALLENGES OF THE TECHNOLOGY

Because evidence-based recommendations call for active learning methods, nurse educators have increased their use of both technology and gaming during learning experiences (Sarker et al., 2021). Ready availability and increasing ease of use of gaming technologies have drastically increased teachers' confidence in their ability to incorporate gaming technology into learning experiences, providing realistic clinical decision making and immediate feedback (Malicki et al, 2020; Xu et al., 2021). Gamification delivers content in a way that is more engaging to students, while providing a break from passive, lecture-based delivery of content (Cvetković et al., 2022; Sarker et al., 2021; Tavares, 2022). Students practice using clinical judgment to answer complex questions within a safe learning environment (Pollio et al., 2021). These activities allow nursing students to take risks in their clinical decision making, receive immediate feedback, and learn from their errors (Brull & Finlayson, 2016; García-Viola et al., 2019; Malicki et al., 2020). This could positively affect future clinical outcomes because it allows students to learn from their errors and improve knowledge without impacting actual nursing care of clients.

Despite the growing trends of gamifying learning in higher education, some nurse educators have been slow to adopt gamification in favor of traditional lecture-based learning (van Gaalen et al., 2021; Xu et al., 2021). Barriers that impede adoption of gamification include the teacher's confidence and perceived competence in using gaming technologies and concerns regarding whether gaming produces useful learning outcomes (Reed, 2020). Structural barriers include a lack of technological resources for gaming or lack of trust in available technology (Cvetković et al., 2022; Reed, 2020). One recurring barrier voiced by faculty members is the lack of time to learn to use various technologies and prepare games for learning (Polly et al., 2021). Another barrier to the use of gamification is the potential cost, often due to many programs' and students' limited financial resources; however, many gamification sites and tools offer free versions (Sánchez-Mena & Martí-Parreño, 2017).

SAMPLE CASE INTEGRATION

Case 1: Kahoot Gaming

Our medical-surgical nursing course implemented pre-/postquizzes into simulation prebriefings and debriefings several years ago to add an element of active learning to solely discussion-based portions of the simulation experience. However, the paper-based quizzes included mostly knowledge-based questions and did little to engage students in preparation for or reflection on the simulation. Students and instructors all agreed a change was needed to improve these quizzes. The medical-surgical teaching team decided to add an element of competition to simulation prebriefing and debriefing quizzes as a way to energize the students and spark their ability to connect simulation learning objectives to course concepts.

The Kahoot quizzing platform was used to create pairs of prebrief/debrief quizzes with five items each for every simulation used in our course. Prebriefing quizzes included items to stimulate thinking about the disease process experienced by the simulated patient and reinforce key concepts prior to the simulation. Debriefing quizzes asked about patient teaching, communication with health care providers, or analysis of patient data in the simulation and were designed to stimulate reflection, thus building clinical judgment. Table 9.1 includes mapping of a course objective to an activity with Kahoot.

Evaluation of the Technology

The relevant clinical content and application/analysis level of the prebriefing and debriefing Kahoot quizzes stimulated more discussion and case analysis during these parts of

TABLE 9.1			
Educational Map: Simulation Prebriefing and Debriefing With Kahoot			
Objective	**Student Population**	**Implementation**	**Evaluation**
Identify alterations in metabolism, glucose regulation, and fluid/electrolyte imbalances.	Prelicensure undergraduate medical-surgical nursing course	Clinical groups of six to eight students compete against each other in two five-question Kahoot quizzes during simulation prebriefing and debriefing sessions.	Course faculty review response statistics following each Kahoot question as formative evaluation and initiate follow-up discussion to clarify muddy points for learners.

our simulation learning experiences. Clinical faculty observed that prebriefing quizzes stimulated excitement and questions about the upcoming simulation and that debriefing quizzes prompted more reflection and analysis of the simulation cases. In addition, our full-time teaching team observed that the Kahoot quizzing provided structure and content for discussion that helped our adjunct clinical faculty teaching simulations in our medical-surgical course, improving the quality and depth of simulation prebriefing and debriefing discussions across all clinical groups.

Case 2: Quiz Show Gaming Platforms

Jeopardy is a well-known television program that has been around for many years. Users are familiar with the components, so this style can lessen some of the anxiety barriers that students experience with something new. Open-source platforms simulating this game show have long been used in classrooms and are often marketed as quiz show games. Quiz show games often utilize software such as Microsoft Excel and PowerPoint that are already installed on classroom computers. Many different specialty templates are available at no cost for instructors to adapt to their course topics. We have integrated quiz show technologies into multiple courses within our undergraduate curriculum to stimulate clinical decision making, help students review concepts, and engage students in active learning. One example of the use of a quiz show has been in a pharmacology course to help students think through the nursing implications of administering medications for perfusion (Table 9.2). Engaging titles assigned to each category included "High Pressure," "Bust the Clots," "Code Situation," "Cheeseburger Cheeseburger," "Off to the Lab," and "Perfusion Potpourri." The quiz show game also included a final category, "Who Knows?" Figure 9.1 shows a quiz show screen.

The students worked together in small groups of six to eight to discuss potential answers to the questions. This prompted collaboration among students, helping them learn from each other as they debated over which answer to choose. Students frequently competed for small prizes available for the winning group. The versatility and adaptability of quiz show games make them ideal for varying class sizes; we have used

TABLE 9.2

Educational Map: Jeopardy Game

Objective	Student Population	Implementation	Evaluation
Apply knowledge of medication administration for perfusion examples	Prelicensure undergraduate pharmacology nursing course	Small groups (number dependent on class size) will collaborate on clinical questions presented through the quiz show game. A leader will provide a final answer from the group.	Formative assessment during the activity to evaluate if students can produce the correct answer. If successful, the instructor will ask follow-up questions to clarify content for the students. If unsuccessful, the instructor will ask what makes the answer incorrect to help students arrive at the correct answer.

them with classes ranging from 25 to 80 students. Moreover, they function well in both in-person and synchronous online learning environments. In addition to playing quiz show games in person, we frequently create and share this style of game with students to use in their independent study groups where they can compete against each other while reviewing content for exams. Figures 9.2 and 9.3 show a typical question and answer screen.

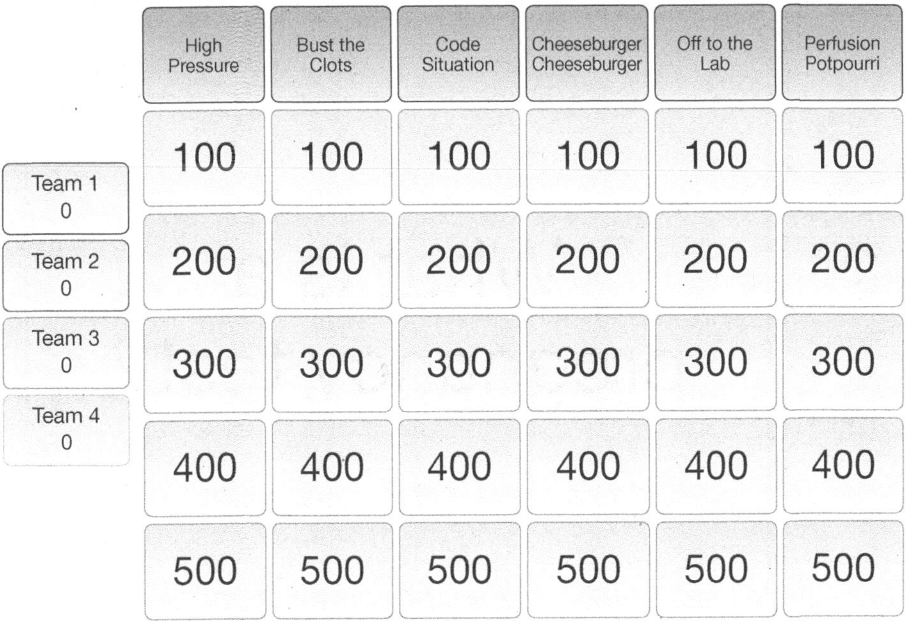

	High Pressure	Bust the Clots	Code Situation	Cheeseburger Cheeseburger	Off to the Lab	Perfusion Potpourri
Team 1 0	100	100	100	100	100	100
Team 2 0	200	200	200	200	200	200
Team 3 0	300	300	300	300	300	300
Team 4 0	400	400	400	400	400	400
	500	500	500	500	500	500

FIGURE 9.1 Quiz Show Main Screen.

> **Team 1** ✗ ✓
> **Team 2** ✗ ✓
> **Team 3** ✗ ✓
> **Team 4** ✗ ✓
>
> # Which prescreening test would be needed for a female prior to beginning treatment for HBP with ACEs or ARBs?

⊕⊖   «   ...

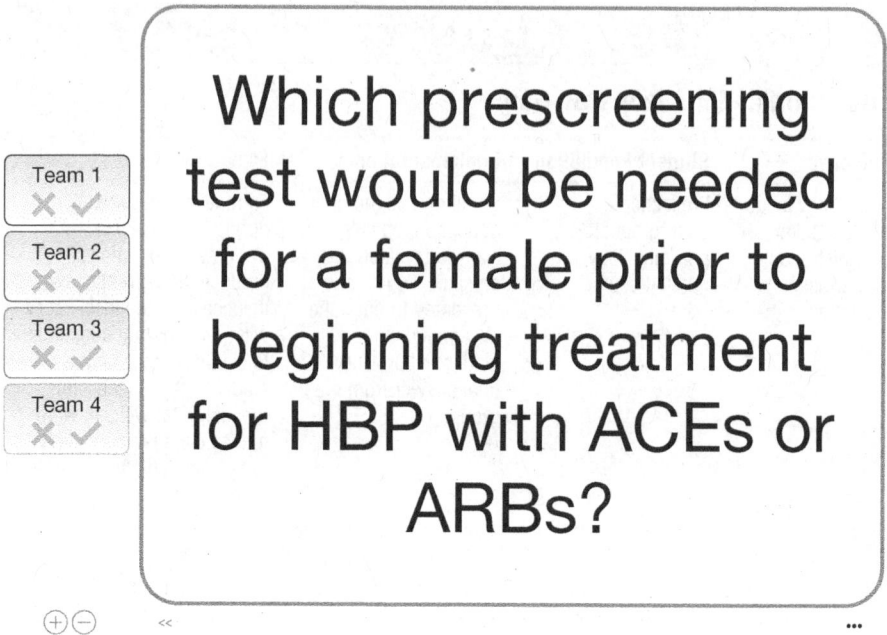

FIGURE 9.2 Pharmacology Perfusion Quiz Show Game: Sample Question Screen. (Please note that "female" in this figure means a person assigned female at birth.)

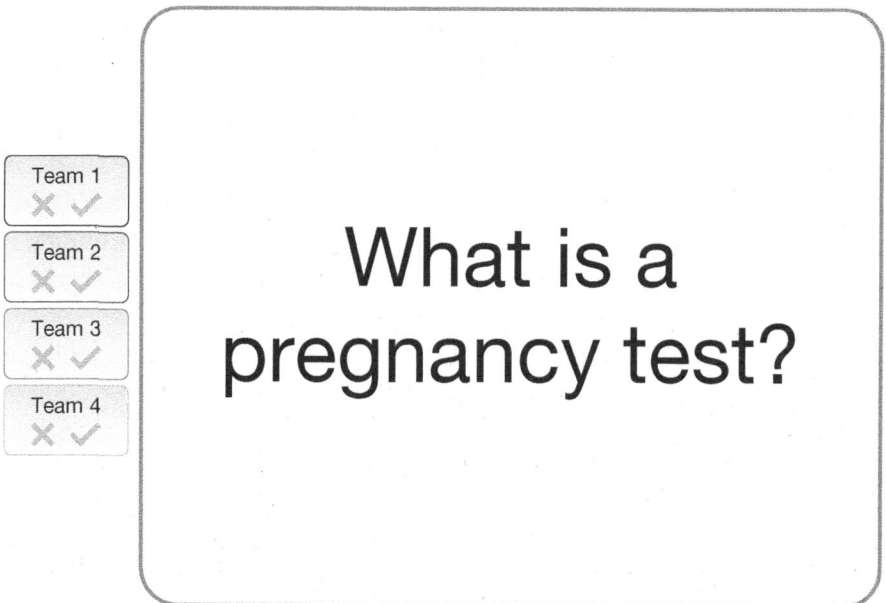

> **Team 1** ✗ ✓
> **Team 2** ✗ ✓
> **Team 3** ✗ ✓
> **Team 4** ✗ ✓
>
> # What is a pregnancy test?

FIGURE 9.3 Pharmacology Perfusion Quiz Show Game: Sample Answer Screen.

Evaluation of the Technology

Content that was taught within the pharmacology for perfusion quiz show helped students make connections between medication effects, laboratory data, and patient assessments. In addition, questions required them to plan patient teaching and anticipate potential adverse effects of medications. Our students enjoyed the entertaining aspects of the technology and being able to apply knowledge in a competitive environment. Students often request we play the Jeopardy theme song while playing the game. Quiz show gamification learning allows students to collaborate on clinical problems in the same way as they would in a health care environment. Guesses at answers often spark additional what-if questions, allowing students to learn from a variety of acceptable responses and formulate additional follow-up questions within their study groups. Students in our program frequently request we create these types of games to help them review for their exams as the questions stimulate them to learn content more deeply.

CONCLUSION

Gamification in nursing education has become increasingly popular in recent years (Meşe & Meşe, 2022; van Gaalen et al., 2021). Increased online components of learning and technology-enabled traditional classrooms have driven many nurse educators to leverage gaming technology to improve student engagement and learning outcomes. Although several barriers exist to gamifying the classroom and other educational environments, both teachers and students have described many benefits to game implementation, including development of clinical judgment, increased enjoyment and engagement, and opportunities for collaborative learning.

References

Brull, S., & Finlayson, S. (2016). Importance of gamification in increasing learning. *The Journal of Continuing Education in Nursing*, *47*(8), 372–375. https://doi.org/10.3928/00220124-20160715-09

Chen, J., & Liang, M. (2022). Play hard, study hard? The influence of gamification on students' study engagement. *Frontiers in Psychology, 13*. https://doi.org/10.3389/fpsyg.2022.994700

Cvetković, B., Arsić, Z., & Cenić, D. (2022). Attitudes of teachers to using information and communication technology in teaching—advantages and obstacles. *International Journal of Cognitive Research in Science, Engineering, and Education, 10*(2). https://doi.org/10.23947/2334-8496-2022-10-2-69-76

García-Viola, A., Garrido-Molina, J. M., Márquez-Hernández, V. V., Granados-Gámez, G., Aguilera-Manrique, G., & Gutiérrez-Puertas, L. (2019). The influence of gamification on decision making in nursing students. *Journal of Nursing Education*, *58*(12), 718–722. https://doi:10.3928/01484834-20191120-07

Khaldi, A., Bouzidi. R., & Nader, F. (2023). Gamification of e-learning in higher education: A systematic literature review. *Smart Learning Environments 10*(1), 1–31. https://doi.org/10.1186/s40561-023-00227-z

Malicki, A., Vergara, F. H., Van de Castle, B., Goyeneche, P., Mann, S., Scott, M. P., Seiler, J., Meneses, M. Z., & Whalen, M. (2020). Gamification in nursing education: An integrative literature review. *Journal of*

Continuing Education in Nursing, 51(11), 509–515. https://doi-org.elib.uah.edu/10.3928/00220124-20201014-07

McEnroe-Petitte, D. M., & Farris, C. (2020). Using gaming as an active teaching strategy in nursing education. *Teaching and Learning in Nursing, 15*(1), 61–65. https://doi.org/10.1016/j.teln.2019.09.002

Meşe, S., & Meşe, C. (2022). Research trends on digital games and gamification in nursing education. *Journal of Computer and Education Research, 10*(20), 734–750. https://doi.org/10.18009/jcer.1175412

Pollio, E. W., Patton, E., Nichols, L. W., & Bowers, D. (2021). Gamification of primary care in a baccalaureate nursing education program. *Nursing Education Perspectives, 44*(2), 126–127. https://doi.org/10.1097/01.nep.0000000000000925

Polly, D., Martin, F., & Guilbaud, T. C. (2021). Examining barriers and desired supports to increase faculty members' use of digital technologies: Perspectives of faculty, staff, and administrators. *Journal of Computing in Higher Education, 33*(1), 135–156. https://doi.org/10.1007/s12528-020-09259-7

Reed, J. E. (2020). Gaming in nursing education: Recent trends and future paths. *Journal of Nursing Education, 59*(7), 375–381. http://dx.doi.org.elib.uah.edu/10.3928/01484834-20200617-04

Sánchez-Mena, A., & Martí-Parreño, J. (2017). Drivers and barriers to adopting gamification: Teachers' perspectives. *Electronic Journal of e-Learning, 15*(5), 434–443. http://files.eric.ed.gov/fulltext/EJ1157970.pdf

Sarker, U., Kanuka, H., Norris, C. M., Raymond, C., Yonge, O., & Davidson, S. (2021). Gamification in nursing literature: An integrative review. *International Journal of Nursing Education Scholarship, 18*(1). https://doi.org/10.1515/ijnes-2020-0081

Shapiro, A. D., Sims-Knight, J. E., O'Rielly, G., Capaldo, P., Pedlow, T., Gordon, L. T., & Monteiro, K. (2017). Clickers can promote fact retention but impede conceptual understanding: The effect of the interaction between clicker use and pedagogy on learning. *Computers & Education, 111*(1), 44–59. https://doi.org/10.1016/j.compedu.2017.03.017

Suh, D., Kim, H., Suh, E., & Kim, H. (2022). The effect of game-based clinical nursing skills mobile application on nursing students. *Computers, Informatics, Nursing, 40*(11), 769–778. https://10.1097/cin.0000000000000865

Tavares, N. (2022). The use and impact of game-based learning on the learning experience and knowledge retention of nursing undergraduate students: A systematic literature review. *Nurse Education Today, 117*, 105484. https://doi.org/10.1016/j.nedt.2022.105484

van Gaalen, A. E. J., Brouwer, J. T., Schönrock-Adema, J., Bouwkamp-Timmer, T., Jaarsma, D., & Georgiadis, J. R. (2021). Gamification of health professions education: A systematic review. *Advances in Health Sciences Education 26*(2), 683–711. https://doi.org/10.1007/s10459-020-10000-3

Wingo, N. P., Roche, C., Baker, N. A., Dunn, D., Jennings, M., Pair, L. S., Somerall, D., Somerall, W. E., White, T., & Willig, J. H. (2019). Playing for bragging rights: A qualitative study of students' perceptions of gamification. *Journal of Nursing Education, 58*(2), 79–85. https://doi.org/10.3928/01484834-20190122-04

Xu, Y., Lau, Y., Cheng, L., & Lau, S. T. (2021). Learning experiences of game-based educational intervention in nursing students: A systematic mixed-studies review. *Nurse Education Today, 107*, 105139. https://doi.org/10.1016/j.nedt.2021.105139

Zehler, A., & Musallam, E. (2021). Game-based learning and nursing students' clinical judgment in postpartum hemorrhage: A pilot study. *The Journal of Nursing Education, 60*(3), 159–164. https://doi.org/10.3928/01484834-20210222-07

10

Polling and Survey Tools

Matthew Byrne, PhD, RN, CNE

Digital technologies have significantly expanded opportunities for faculty to perform assessments and evaluations in both online and face-to-face environments. Polling and survey software have many uses but are particularly valuable as an option for digital formative assessment (DFA), in which faculty monitor progress in student learning and improve instruction. Polling and survey tools vary in terms of the kinds of questions that can be asked, the kinds of responses that can be delivered, integration with other technologies such as presentation software, and analysis options. The large variety of often free polling and survey software creates a wide range of uses and benefits for faculty and students alike.

DESCRIPTION OF THE TECHNOLOGY

At its most basic, polling and survey software allow for one or more sequences of prompt and response using multiple-choice, true/false, multiselect, and/or free text formatted questions. In most cases, faculty are inquiring about some aspect of student learning or seeking feedback about the learning that is underway. Polling and survey software are often specifically used as part of a classroom assessment technique (CAT) to gather DFA data. Formative assessments, digital or otherwise, are often ungraded or low stakes and can give faculty a sense of how they might need to adjust their teaching and student progress toward learning outcomes.

The choice of polling and survey software is driven by how, why, and when faculty may want to use it. For example, faculty may ask themselves if they want to regularly use this software versus for one particular teaching technique in a given class or if they want to use it primarily for engaging students versus trying to get more concrete metrics about student learning. The software may be designed for asynchronous (e.g., SurveyMonkey) or synchronous (e.g., Slido) situations. Synchronous use allows for teaching and DFA to occur simultaneously. Faculty can develop prompts using downloaded desktop software, stand-alone smartphone applications, or websites (e.g., VoxVote, GoSoapBox). Historically, clicker hardware was required for student responses with some applications, but now web or smartphone applications reduce the potential barrier of hardware, cost, and ease of use (e.g., Echo360). Increasingly, polling and survey tools are directly integrated into videoconferencing software or course management systems

(CMS). For example, all commercial CMS have test and quiz capabilities with basic question and answer functions with varying levels of sophistication that can also be repurposed to allow for DFA, typically in an asynchronous context. Videoconferencing systems, such as Webex, Google Meet, and Zoom, have built-in survey tools designed for synchronous data collection. Presentation software also may have integrated options (e.g., Mentimeter, AhaSlides, and Google Slides have built-in digital polling that allows for real-time responses, and several software vendors can directly integrate into presentation applications such as PowerPoint, including Poll Everywhere, Vevox, and ClassPoint).

Student responses are a key part of what make polling and survey software valuable for students and faculty alike. Software options may be differentiated by functional options, such as more diverse question formatting (e.g., videos or images vs plain text). When used in a synchronous learning environment, real-time presentation of data can be valuable for students and faculty. Response data can also be anonymous or linked to respondents depending on the software selected and available settings. A wide range of postsurvey analytics and data downloads may be available, particularly for software options that are more typically marketed as survey applications, such as Google Forms, Office 365 Forms, SurveyPlanet, SogoSurvey, and commercial tools such as Qualtrics and SurveyMonkey. More sophisticated options can drive secondary actions, such as follow-up questions based on scoring, more complex visual analytics (e.g., visual presentations such as Word clouds), and automated feedback options based on responses (e.g., Classflow, Edulastic).

EVIDENCE-BASED ADVANTAGES AND CHALLENGES OF THE TECHNOLOGY

The evidence base for the use of DFA is mixed partially because most of the research occurs in K-12 settings and there are issues with the quality and quantity of studies (Kaya-Capocci et al., 2022; Morris et al., 2021). The evidence base supporting the use of polling and survey software varies also by the intended use, such as specific studies that have looked at game-based learning (gamification). In general, survey and polling tools create value for learning when applied as part of active learning strategies and through provision of formative assessment data.

Kaya-Capocci et al. (2022) created a formative assessment implementation framework that included categories of typical software functional options, which in turn allowed for a set of formative assessment strategies. The strategies included sharing learning intentions and success criteria, questioning and discussion, feedback, and peer and self-assessment. These strategies are then carried out using the technical functions typical of polling and survey tools, which can be used individually or in combination, including:

▸ Sending and displaying assessment data, often in a dashboard or visually presented to all learners

▸ Processing and analyzing of the data, often in comparison to a set standard

▸ Provision of an interactive environment where learners and faculty can all work collaboratively

An implementation framework may be helpful given the many factors that must be considered for planning and implementation as well as the many contexts and timing of use. In the context of prelearning, polling and survey software can be used for diagnostic evaluations or formative assessments. At the beginning of a course, they may be used for baseline knowledge assessments or to gather information about the learners themselves, such as their learning preferences and style, goals and interests, and readiness to learn (González-Gómez et al., 2020; Yavuzalp & Bahcivan, 2021). During synchronous sessions, data can be used as a more traditional formative assessment (CAT) to get a sense of how students are progressing and to help faculty adjust the pace or content depth (Hanson & Florestano, 2020). They might also be used as informal icebreakers and get-to-know-you activities early on in a course or at the start of a class session.

Several benefits have been investigated and identified for both faculty and learners. They include:

> Student learning and understanding of content (Demeke, 2023; Díez-Pascual & García Díaz, 2020; González-Gómez et al., 2020)

> Student motivation (Çekiç & Bakla, 2021; Díez-Pascual & García Díaz, 2020; González-Gómez et al., 2020)

> Reduction in dispositional barriers to learning, such as introversion, shyness, anxiety, or low self-efficacy (Howell et al., 2023)

> Student engagement, attention, and participation (Çekiç & Bakla, 2021; Demeke, 2023)

> Student self-evaluation (Díez-Pascual & García Díaz, 2020)

> Positive student attitude (Díez-Pascual & García Díaz, 2020)

> Greater faculty presence (Çekiç & Bakla, 2021; Howell et al., 2023)

> Faculty feedback on learning progress and for evaluation data (Çekiç & Bakla, 2021; Li & van Lieu, 2018; O'Leary et al., 2018)

Polling and survey tools are ideal for active learning strategies (Demeke, 2023), including game-based learning (gamification). Arruzza and Chau (2021) reported on the use of gamification in health science programs, with a concentration of studies for nursing, and found positive outcomes that included knowledge acquisition, student satisfaction, and motivation. Several polling and survey tools can cross-functionally act as gamification platforms. Competition as a motivator is one such technique that can be leveraged with software such as Kahoot, Quizizz, Triventy, Classflow, and Nearpod, in which points or badges are awarded and result dashboards are visible to students.

Çekiç & Bakla (2021) did a large-scale review of the features of 14 DFA applications and noted that student progress data was crucial to identifying problems and adjusting teaching as needed. As an example, a quick DFA called "muddiest point" is often used by faculty to get a sense of what content or concepts students may be struggling with so faculty can review or remediate accordingly (Li & van Lieu, 2018; Mackos & Tornwall, 2021). These adjustments can be made in real time and increase student success, particularly when feedback can be personalized to the student. Survey and polling tools can also be used for terminal points in learning, such as at the end of a class session, chunk of content, or at the end of the course itself.

Despite the benefits of polling and survey tools, particularly for formative assessments, faculty need to be aware of challenges when considering adoption and implementation. For synchronous software options it may be difficult for faculty to lecture or facilitate learning while also monitoring feedback and responses, especially if there is a high volume of student messages. Large courses may also limit individualization or quick pattern analysis unless prompts are properly structured (Çekiç & Bakla, 2021). For example, the built-in Google Slide feedback is free text; in a big class, this could get overwhelming to follow so more structured prompts within Google Forms might be better suited to courses with a large number of students. Faculty need to be aware of the risk for incivilities or inappropriate responses when there are anonymous, open-ended response options. Digital literacy, software compatibility with devices, data security, privacy, and technology access may also be issues for both students and faculty to consider when selecting and implementing software (Demeke, 2023). Analysis of the ways students can participate (e.g., compatibility with smartphone operating systems as well as web-based participation) may reduce the likelihood of technology barriers. Many of the applications allow students to be respondents at no cost, and educator free trials can reduce cost as a barrier for several applications. Lastly, if software is overused, burnout and loss of novelty with the technology can occur (Arruzza & Chau, 2021).

SAMPLE CASE INTEGRATION

Due to a large snowstorm, an undergraduate baccalaureate nursing faculty needed to quickly convert an in-class learning session focused on hospice care into a synchronized hybrid learning experience. About half of the students who lived on campus were in the classroom, and the other half were online via Google Meet. All students joined Google Meet to participate in the planned collaborative online learning activities. The faculty divided all students into teams of approximately four each, with the in-class students meeting face to face and virtual students divided into digital breakout rooms. The students were all provided with different unfolding case studies that would be revealed to students based on how they responded to questions on a Google Form. The students used Google's Jamboard to collaboratively add signs/symptoms, medications, and nursing interventions based on prompts and scenarios within the unfolding case study. The faculty checked on student progress by reviewing and commenting on Google Jamboards, using the polling feature within Google Meet, and monitoring Google Form data that showed student progress in the unfolding case study based on the quantity of questions the student teams had answered. Table 10.1 includes how course objectives match to the technology integration.

EVALUATION OF THE TECHNOLOGY

Evaluation of the technology must be done from both student and faculty perspectives. In both cases, the technology must have a high degree of usability in terms of learning how to use it, ease of achieving the goals of its use, and effectiveness primarily for DFA. Faculty may desire specific sets of functionalities based on the teaching/learning context. In the case study earlier, there may be benefits to staying within the Google suite of tools to reduce sign-ins and because of student familiarity with navigation and function. The faculty in this case study found a fit because they wanted a dynamic, active learning option that allowed for simultaneous engagement with online and face-to-face learners. A DFA integrated into the presentation software (Google Slides) that could be used on a

TABLE 10.1

Educational Map: Polling Tool

Course Objectives	Student Population	Implementation	Evaluation
Identify signs and symptoms of impending patient death	Undergraduate baccalaureate nursing students	Students will use their digital Jamboard to brainstorm by putting one individual sign or symptom on each digital sticky note.	Students will have a complete and accurate list of signs and symptoms.
Describe priority nursing next steps when a patient condition changes	Undergraduate baccalaureate nursing students	Students will use Google Forms survey software to advance the case study and for feedback on their decisions related to priorities of care.	Students will have an accurate list of nursing actions and articulate the rationale for why; they will receive feedback through responses embedded in Google Forms.
Apply pharmacological plan of care based on standing orders and context of care	Undergraduate baccalaureate nursing students	Students will use the digital sticky notes to brainstorm pharmacological options based on case study standing orders and readings for the class session.	Students accurately match medications to the context of care, such as nausea or pain.

personal computer made the most sense. One gap for faculty in this scenario is a more detailed assessment of individual student participation, which might have made Google Docs a better fit given its participation history and versioning features, making it a better choice than Jamboard.

Ultimately the fit of the application to the context is critical with consideration of factors, such as cost, usability, requirements for respondent analytics, and assessment scenario, which help faculty select the best options. Çekiç & Bakla (2021) focused on evaluation in their examination of 14 DFA applications and specifically looked at accessibility, performance monitoring, scoring, feedback, platforms, devices, quizzing, gamification, practicality, and cost. Accessibility, particularly for screen readers, and usability were the focus of a review by Rybin Koob et al. (2022). They found Mentimeter to be most accessible, but all the tools, which also included Kahoot! Padlet, Jamboard, and Poll Everywhere, had severe or significant accessibility concerns in the versions analyzed at that time. Ultimately, any software, including polling and survey tools, which have a high degree of accessibility, will benefit all learners, not just those with diagnosed or even undiagnosed disabilities. Formalized technology evaluation rubrics may also help faculty compare two or more different options or guide evaluation after use of the technology to determine fit for future learning experiences.

CONCLUSION

Polling and survey applications have the potential to expand traditional assessment and measurement strategies that can benefit both formative and summative evaluation. The use of these applications, which are in many cases low or no cost, have several benefits to students and faculty alike in areas such as student engagement, faculty presence, and more timely feedback cycle. Faculty need to carefully evaluate many aspects of the fit of technology to the learners, type of learning experience, and educational needs.

References

Arruzza, E., & Chau, M. (2021). A scoping review of randomised controlled trials to assess the value of gamification in the higher education of health science students. *Journal of Medical Imaging and Radiation Sciences, 52*(1), 137–146. https://doi.org/10.1016/j.jmir.2020.10.003

Çekiç, A., & Bakla, A. (2021). A review of digital formative assessment applications: Features and future directions. *International Online Journal of Education and Teaching, 8*(3), 1459–1485.

Demeke, W. (2023). Adoption and use of smart devices as clickers in classrooms in higher education. *Computer Applications in Engineering Education, 31*(4), 963–982. https://doi.org/10.1002/cae.22617

Díez-Pascual, A. M., & García Díaz, M. P. G. (2020). Audience response software as a learning tool in university courses. *Education Sciences, 10*(12), 350. https://doi.org/10.3390/educsci10120350

González-Gómez, D., Jeong, J. S., Cañada-Cañada, F., & Cañada-Cañada, F. (2020). Examining the effect of an online formative assessment tool (OFAT) of students' motivation and achievement for a university science education. *Journal of Baltic Science Education, 19*(3), 401–414. https://doi.org/10.33225/jbse/20.19.401

Hanson, J. M., & Florestano, M. (2020). Classroom assessment techniques: A critical component for effective instruction. *New Directions for Teaching & Learning, 164*, 49–56. https://doi.org/10.1002/tl.20423

Howell, S. L., Johnson, M. C., & Hansen, J. C. (2023). The innovative use of technological tools (the ABCs and Ps) to help adult learners decrease transactional distance and increase learning presence. *Adult Learning, 34*(3). https://doi.org/10.1177/10451595221149768

Kaya-Capocci, S., O'Leary, M., & Costello, E. (2022). Towards a framework to support the implementation of digital formative assessment in higher education. *Education Sciences, 12*(11), 11. https://doi.org/10.3390/educsci12110823

Li, M., & van Lieu, S. (2018). Traditional and online faculty members' use of classroom assessment technique (CATs): A mixed-method study. *Journal of Instructional Research, 7*, 90–99.

Mackos, A., & Tornwall, J. (2021). Muddiest points assessment to increase understanding in a large-enrollment course. *Nurse Educator, 46*(1), 42–42. https://doi.org/10.1097/NNE.0000000000000869

Morris, R., Perry, T., & Wardle, L. (2021). Formative assessment and feedback for learning in higher education: A systematic review. *Review of Education, 9*(3), e3292. https://doi.org/10.1002/rev3.3292

O'Leary, M., Scully, D., Karakolidis, A., & Pitsia, V. (2018). The state-of-the-art in digital technology-based assessment. *European Journal of Education, 53*(2), 160–175. https://doi.org/10.1111/ejed.12271

Rybin Koob, A., Ibacache Oliva, K. S., Williamson, M., Lamont-Manfre, M., Hugen, A., & Dickerson, A. (2022). Tech tools in pandemic-transformed information literacy instruction: Pushing for digital accessibility. *Information Technology & Libraries, 41*(4), 1–32. https://doi.org/10.6017/ital.v41i4.15383

Yavuzalp, N., & Bahcivan, E. (2021). A structural equation modeling analysis of relationships among university students' readiness for e-learning, self-regulation skills, satisfaction, and academic achievement. *Research and Practice in Technology Enhanced Learning, 16*(1), 15. https://doi.org/10.1186/s41039-021-00162-y

11

Adaptive Testing-Based Formative Assessment

Kevin Mazor, PhD

Adaptive testing-based formative assessments (e.g., quizzes or examinations) represent a type of formative evaluation that aims to improve the efficacy of testing-based formative assessments by identifying a student's strengths and weaknesses and then adapting the questions and difficulty of the assessments to those characteristics (Fontaine et al., 2019). This chapter will focus on the use of testing-based assessments in nursing education. A note on terminology: During this chapter whenever the term *assessment* is used, it can be assumed that it represents a testing-based assessment. In addition, unless specifically noted, adaptive and nonadaptive assessments describe testing-based formative assessments.

DESCRIPTION OF THE TECHNOLOGY

Adaptive assessments tailor exam questions in real time to the ability of each individual test taker based on data characterizing the student's strengths and weaknesses (Sharma et al., 2017). It is often dependent on computer-based technology (i.e., computerized adaptive testing). Two main methods can be used to implement an adaptive assessment: designed adaptive assessments and algorithmic adaptive assessments. In designed adaptive assessments, the educator determines how the assessment will react to the student's data. This method uses a simple if-then approach, wherein student performance results in a standard outcome that is consistent for all students. For example, if a student answers a question incorrectly, then the student will be exposed to a second question on the same topic; by contrast, if a student answers a question correctly, then the student will progress to the next topic. Designed adaptive assessments can be created by the educator using survey programs that contain advanced flow rules or conditions such as Qualtrics (https://www.qualtrics.com) and Jotform (https://www.jotform.com).

In algorithmic adaptive assessments, an algorithm is used to adjust the assessment based on additional data from the student. Algorithmic assessments often rely on student-level data, including past performance or time spent on questions, as well as more advanced techniques, such as artificial intelligence or natural language processing. As a result, each student can receive a completely unique assessment based on individual needs and performance (Fontaine et al., 2019). Examples of algorithmic assessments include PrepU by thePoint, Elsevier Adaptive Quizzing, and the ATI Learning System 3.0.

EVIDENCE-BASED ADVANTAGES AND CHALLENGES OF THE TECHNOLOGY

Fundamentally, testing has been viewed as primarily a means of summative assessment. However, there is some evidence that, during testing, a student is required to retrieve information learned and respond to any retrieval errors, thereby leading to improved understanding of the topic and improved formative assessment. This phenomenon is known as the testing effect (Heitmann et al., 2018). Multiple studies have shown the benefits of testing-based formative assessments for retrieval-enhanced learning compared to other studying and testing modalities (Polack & Miller, 2022; Sartain & Wright, 2021; Yang et al., 2019; Yang et al., 2021). A recent systematic review and meta-analysis reported that short-answer and multiple-choice questions are effective at enhancing learning; however, multiple-choice questions may be more effective than short-answer questions as additional feedback can be obtained through answering each question (Yang et al., 2021). Additionally, they found that:

▸ Learning is enhanced when the format of the formative assessment matches the format of the summative assessment.

▸ The more times that a topic is covered in the formative assessment, the greater effect that it has on learning; however, testing can also enhance the learning of other topics that are not covered on the formative assessment.

▸ A higher level of difficulty on the formative assessment can enhance learning, especially when the summative assessment is set at a lower level of difficulty.

▸ Taking the formative assessment during or outside of the classroom offers benefits, but in-class assessments may have a marginally enhanced effect on learning compared to out-of-class assessments.

Advantages/Strengths of Adaptive Assessments

The National Council Licensure Examination for Registered Nurses (NCLEX-RN) transitioned to a computerized adaptive format in 1994 (National Council of State Boards of Nursing [NCSBN], 2014) and in 2023 launched the next-generation NCLEX exam (NCSBN, 2023). Nursing programs frequently incorporate adaptive assessments into their classrooms to provide students with practice in this format to enhance their preparation for and performance on the NCLEX-RN. Cox-Davenport and Phelan (2015) observed that increased usage of an adaptive assessment program correlated with higher mastery levels, indicating improved knowledge, on the NCLEX-RN. However, these authors reported that, because of the institution's high pass rate and the pass/fail nature of the NCLEX-RN, wider comparison between the adaptive assessment and licensure examination pass rates were inconclusive. Pence and Wood (2018) also demonstrated a reduction in NCLEX-RN failure rates from 16.16 percent to 1.05 percent after introducing an adaptive assessment with NCLEX-RN–style questions (Pence & Wood, 2018). Similarly, Presti and Sanko (2019) reported increased NCLEX-RN pass rates and improved performance on standardized exit examinations following the addition of an adaptive assessment into their capstone adult health course.

Adaptive assessments also benefit students in the classroom environment. Austin et al. (2021) found that performance on standardized end-of-course examinations correlated with the number of adaptive assessments taken and the level of mastery demonstrated on the adaptive assessment program. Similarly, Gupta et al. (2020) reported that students utilizing the assessment program outperformed those who did not on unit and final examinations. They also reported that taking four or more adaptive assessments showed improved final examination performance (Gupta et al., 2020). Furthermore, Heitmann et al. (2018) conducted a controlled laboratory study demonstrating that adaptive assessments yielded superior posttest performance compared to both nonadaptive assessments and focused studying.

Students generally respond positively to adaptive assessments, acknowledging their benefits in exam preparation, the importance of features such as mastery levels in evaluating knowledge, and their effectiveness in strengthening areas of lesser understanding (Gupta et al., 2020; Parcell et al., 2022; Simon-Campbell & Phelan, 2016).

Challenges/Weaknesses of Adaptive Assessments

While adaptive assessments offer potential benefits in adapting to the learning needs of individual learners, current research yields mixed results regarding whether these benefits contribute to learning beyond the testing effect. Heitmann et al. (2018) demonstrated an additional advantage with assessments that adjusted question difficulty based on student performance compared to a control group that received a standard series of questions with increasing difficulty; however, other studies have shown no additional effect of adaptive assessments compared to well-matched nonadaptive controls. Griff and Matter (2013) found no difference in a pre- versus posttest analysis or overall course grades when comparing an adaptive assessment program to instructor-selected questions from the same company's test bank. It is worth noting that this study involved six institutions across the United States, with two institutions showing a potential additional benefit from the adaptive assessments, suggesting a possible role played by the institution or instructor. Kolpikova et al. (2019) similarly found no impact of adaptive assessments covering preclass readings on class preparedness or exam performance, compared to a control group receiving the same number of questions in a nonadaptive format; however, students using the adaptive assessment system perceived a slight increase in the value of preclass reading assessments compared to those using the nonadaptive system.

Algorithmic adaptive assessments require extensive knowledge of various topics such as computer science, artificial intelligence, and natural language processing. Incorporating these assessments into a class or program often relies on the use of third-party systems and can impose additional financial burdens on institutions or students. Moreover, the testing effect works best when testing-based formative assessments align closely with the course material and summative assessments, making algorithmic adaptive assessments less applicable in courses that deviate from the same education system as the adaptive assessment program.

Designed adaptive assessments offer the advantage of tailoring to course outcomes and can be created using commonly available and free survey programs such as Qualtrics (https://www.qualtrics.com) and Jotform (https://www.jotform.com); however, this approach requires instructors to invest additional time in creating the assessments and may not offer the same level of complexity and data availability provided by third-party algorithmic adaptive assessment programs.

SAMPLE CASE INTEGRATION

The examples described here provide effective methods from the literature on how to incorporate adaptive assessments into the classroom. They describe a framework on how adaptive or designed assessments can be used to enhance student learning. In general, when incorporating adaptive assessments into a class, care should be made to ensure the assessments have two key characteristics:

➤ The questions on the assessments are closely related to the course content. These questions can be written by the educator or from the same publisher as other resources used in the class.

➤ They must be formative in nature. If they are incorporated into the final course outcomes, it should be based on some level of completion or mastery where students always have the option to answer more questions to achieve the desired outcome.

Case 1

Presti and Sanko (2019) proposed a method for integrating adaptive assessments into an in-person nursing course, which is easily adapted for online courses. The researchers introduced an algorithmic adaptive assessment program in a senior-level adult health nursing course. Prior to the start of the course, students took a standardized diagnostic examination to identify areas in which their knowledge could be improved. These data were then utilized to determine the topics that the adaptive assessments would cover.

The adaptive assessments consisted of three parts: (1) three assessments targeting the students' lowest scoring individual topics, (2) three assessments focusing on the lowest scoring topics for the entire class, and (3) three assessments covering general topics. To successfully complete the assignments, students were required to achieve a mastery level of two (out of three), and those who reached this mastery level answered between 75 and 90 questions per week. In cases where students could not meet the designated mastery level, they could still earn credit by answering 100 questions on the topic per week.

To evaluate the effectiveness of the adaptive assessments, a chi-squared analysis was conducted to compare the performance of students who received the curriculum with assessments (three sections) to those who did not (one section) on an end-of-program exit examination. While this approach employed a potentially problematic no-assessment control group, the use of a diagnostic pretest to personalize the adaptive assessments proved to be an effective strategy. Moreover, this approach can be easily adapted to transform nonadaptive assessments into adaptive assessments by assigning nonadaptive assessments to individual students based on their diagnostic pretest results (Presti & Sanko, 2019).

Case 2

Heitmann et al. (2018) presented an innovative approach to designing adaptive assessments using short-answer questions. The study took place in a laboratory setting, with the goal of evaluating the effectiveness of different study techniques. The study participants first took a pretest to establish their baseline knowledge and then watched an e-lecture consisting of 26 slides. Following the lecture, the participants engaged in 80 minutes of studying using one of four techniques: (1) testing-based adaptive assessment, (2) testing-based nonadaptive assessment, (3) note-taking, or (4) focused note-taking. In the testing-based assessment conditions, students completed short-answer questions and self-evaluated their responses based on provided feedback. The adaptive assessment then adjusted the difficulty of the subsequent questions based on the students' self-evaluated scores. If the score was below 50 percent, then the following question would be less challenging; scores between 50 and 85 percent led to questions of similar difficulty, and scores above 85 percent prompted the presentation of more difficult questions. The nonadaptive assessment continued on to the next question regardless of student performance. The participants were assessed with a posttest one week later to measure their retention and learning outcomes. The researchers evaluated the effect sizes between each study technique using partial eta-squared analysis (Heitmann et al., 2018).

EVALUATION OF THE TECHNOLOGY

The effectiveness of adaptive assessments has been evaluated using various methods. Retrospective studies have examined the impact of implementing an adaptive assessment system by correlating performance or usage of the adaptive assessment with instructor-designed or standardized assessments, such as the NCLEX-RN (Austin et al., 2021; Parcell et al., 2022; Pence & Wood, 2018). However, randomized and nonrandomized experiments face challenges in establishing effective control groups. Because of the demonstrated effectiveness of the testing effect in improving knowledge and course performance, it may be considered unethical to use a no-assessment condition as a control. Furthermore, using a no-assessment control group limits the ability to differentiate the specific contributions of the adaptive nature of the assessment from the assessment itself (Gupta et al., 2020; Presti & Sanko, 2019; Sartain & Wright, 2021; Simon-Campbell & Phelan, 2016). To address this, controls can be designed where nonadaptive assessments are matched to adaptive assessments based on question number or time taken to complete the assessment (Griff & Matter, 2013; Heitmann et al., 2018; Kolpikova et al., 2019). Effectiveness of control experiments can be assessed similarly to retrospective studies, where adaptive assessment usages or performance is correlated to course outcomes. In addition, a pre-/postanalysis, wherein students are given the same assessment at the beginning and end of the course, can also be an effective method to evaluate controlled experiments (Griff & Matter, 2013; Heitmann et al., 2018).

CONCLUSION

The testing effect has been well established to enhance student learning. Adaptive testing-based formative assessments have the potential to individualize the testing effect to each student and have been shown to increase performance when used to help students prepare for standardized examinations such as the NCLEX-RN. However, whether adaptive assessments provide any additional benefit over nonadaptive assessments is not clear, suggesting that the reliance on third-party programs for algorithmic adaptive assessments, or the time and expertise required to create designed adaptive assessments, may not provide additional benefit over the simpler nonadaptive formative assessments.

References

Austin, E. N., Henson, A. P., Kim, H. J., Ogle, K. T., & Park, H. (2021). Analysis of computer adaptive testing in a pathopharmacology course. *Journal of Nursing Education, 60*(3), 155–158. https://doi.org/10.3928/01484834-20210222-06

Cox-Davenport, R. A., & Phelan, J. C. (2015). Laying the groundwork for NCLEX success: An exploration of adaptive quizzing as an examination preparation method. *Computers, Informatics, Nursing, 33*(5), 208–215. https://doi.org/10.1097/CIN.0000000000000140

Fontaine, G., Cossette, S., Maheu-Cadotte, M.-A., Mailhot, T., Deschênes, M.-F., Mathieu-Dupuis, G., Côté, J., Gagnon, M.-P., & Dubé, V. (2019). Efficacy of adaptive e-learning for health professionals and students: A systematic review and meta-analysis. *BMJ Open, 9*(8), e025252. https://doi.org/10.1136/bmjopen-2018-025252

Griff, E. R., & Matter, S. F. (2013). Evaluation of an adaptive online learning system. *British Journal of Educational Technology, 44*(1), 170–176. https://doi.org/10.1111/j.1467-8535.2012.01300.x

Gupta, S., Ojeh, N., Sa, B., Majumder, M. A. A., Singh, K., & Adams, O. P. (2020). Use of an adaptive e-learning platform as a formative assessment tool in the cardiovascular system course component of an MBBS programme. *Advances in Medical Education and Practice, 11*, 989–996. https://doi.org/10.2147/AMEP.S267834

Heitmann, S., Grund, A., Berthold, K., Fries, S., & Roelle, J. (2018). Testing is more desirable when it is adaptive and still desirable when compared to note-taking. *Frontiers in Psychology, 9*, 2596. https://doi.org/10.3389/fpsyg.2018.02596

Kolpikova, E. P., Chen, D. C., & Doherty, J. H. (2019). Does the format of preclass reading quizzes matter? An evaluation of traditional and gamified, adaptive preclass reading quizzes. *CBE—Life Sciences Education, 18*(4), ar52. https://doi.org/10.1187/cbe.19-05-0098

National Council of State Boards of Nursing. (2014). Pencils down, booklets closed. The evolution of the NCLEX: 20 years as a computer adaptive exam. https://ncsbn.org/public-files/InFocus_Spring2014.pdf

National Council of State Boards of Nursing. (2023). NCSBN launches next generation NCLEX. https://www.ncsbn.org/news/ncsbn-launches-next-generation-nclex-exam

Parcell, H., Morton, K., Froble, D., & Sheaves, C. (2022). Evaluating the effect of pre-exam adaptive quizzing on nursing student exam scores. *Nursing Education Perspectives, 43*(6), e100–e102. https://doi.org/10.1097/01.NEP.0000000000000988

Pence, J., & Wood, F. (2018). Using computer-adaptive quizzing as a tool for national council licensure examination success. *Nursing Education Perspectives, 39*(3), 164–166. https://doi.org/10.1097/01.NEP.0000000000000289

Polack, C. W., & Miller, R. R. (2022). Testing improves performance as well as assesses learning: A review of the testing effect with implications for models of learning. *Journal of Experimental Psychology: Animal Learning and Cognition*, *48*(3), 222–241. https://doi.org/10.1037/xan0000323

Presti, C. R., & Sanko, J. S. (2019). Adaptive quizzing improves end-of-program exit examination scores. *Nurse Educator*, *44*(3), 151–153. https://doi.org/10.1097/NNE.0000000000000566

Sartain, A. F., & Wright, V. H. (2021). The effects of frequent quizzing on exam scores in a baccalaureate nursing course. *Nursing Education Perspectives*, *42*(1), 39–40. https://doi.org/10.1097/01.NEP.0000000000000623

Sharma, N., Doherty, I., & Dong, C. (2017). Adaptive learning in medical education: The final piece of technology enhanced learning? *The Ulster Medical Journal*, *86*(3), 198–200.

Simon-Campbell, E., & Phelan, J. (2016). Effectiveness of an adaptive quizzing system as an institutional-wide strategy to improve student learning and retention. *Nurse Educator*, *41*(5), 246–251. https://doi.org/10.1097/NNE.0000000000000258

Yang, B. W., Razo, J., & Persky, A. M. (2019). Using testing as a learning tool. *American Journal of Pharmaceutical Education*, *83*(9), 7324. https://doi.org/10.5688/ajpe7324

Yang, C., Luo, L., Vadillo, M. A., Yu, R., & Shanks, D. R. (2021). Testing (quizzing) boosts classroom learning: A systematic and meta-analytic review. *Psychological Bulletin*, *147*(4), 399–435. https://doi.org/10.1037/bul0000309

12

Integrating Video Technology into Nursing Education

Yeyin Yi, DNP, APRN

In nursing education, video technology is a well-established multimedia form (Dinmore, 2019; Musa et al., 2021). Considerable advancement in technology initiated a call by the American Association of Colleges of Nursing (2019) and the National League for Nursing (2015) to innovate teaching and learning strategies across nursing programs in the United States. Faster internet speeds, increased affordability, and advanced multimedia production (e.g., computers, smart portable devices) collectively transformed the use of video technology in the classroom far beyond its traditional didactic expectations (Arkenback, 2023; Dinmore, 2019; Gazza et al., 2021). Widespread video streaming and cloud-based computing also helped broaden the confines of teaching nursing theory and clinical practice from within the classroom to a greater range of pedagogical modalities that promoted flexibility and accessibility (Dinmore, 2019; Huang et al., 2019). Furthermore, rapid and sustained growth of online prelicensure and graduate-level nursing programs prompted a renewed reliance on video technology to deliver their respective core course components and essentials (Belt & Lowenthal, 2021; Forbes et al., 2016; Gazza et al., 2021; Jonassen & Yarbrough, 2021; Purpora & Prion, 2018; Smith et al., 2022; Wolf, 2018).

Advancements in video technology influenced the emergence of nursing simulation and augmented nursing pedagogical patterns that aim to integrate and contextualize the amalgamation of nursing fundamentals, technical skills, and application (Arkenback, 2023; Belt & Lowenthal, 2021; Dinmore, 2019; Wolf, 2018). Although video technology in education has advanced and evolved in recent years because of technological modernizations, the function and use of video in nursing education predominantly remain in three sustained overarching themes: (1) delivery of lectures, (2) assessment and feedback of clinical skills and practice, and (3) facilitation of engagement and communication (Arkenback, 2023; Belt & Lowenthal, 2021; Clerkin et al., 2022; Dodson, 2023; Forbes et al., 2016; Purpora & Prion, 2018).

DESCRIPTION OF THE TECHNOLOGY

The most recognizable use of video technology in nursing education is the delivery and distribution of lecture content. This is especially true in online nursing programs where

TABLE 12.1

Options for Cloud-Based Video Technology Software

Asynchronous	Synchronous	Asynchronous or Synchronous
Camtasia	Cisco Webex	Google Meet
Kaltura	Go To Meeting	Microsoft Teams
Learning management system (LMS)		Zoom
Microsoft PowerPoint		
OBS Studio		
Panopto		
VoiceThread		

video is the primary means to transfer knowledge from faculty to students either synchronously or asynchronously. Traditionally, didactic course materials were recorded using one's built-in or auxiliary plug-in camera and microphone, which were directly accessed and processed by software programs (e.g., Microsoft PowerPoint) or embedded within a learning management system (LMS) (Krautscheid, 2021; Toulouse, 2020). Today, a plethora of software programs that record and edit audiovisual recordings of on-screen content using personal computers and smart devices is readily available in part due to increased broadband access and ongoing application development (Table 12.1) (Belt & Lowenthal, 2021).

Screen capture software (e.g., Camtasia, Panopto, PowerPoint, Kaltura) enable instructors to concurrently record on-screen content and audio commentary in real time (i.e., slides, images, documents). The addition of a small-scale video of the instructor's face or upper body seen picture in picture (e.g., talking head) enhances viewer connection and heightens social presence. Literature indicates that videos presented in this way are as effective as traditional lectures and surpass voice-over-only formats in engagement (Belt & Lowenthal, 2021; Garcia & Yousef, 2023). While typically utilized in asynchronous contexts, the mechanism is also applicable in synchronous settings (i.e., videoconferences).

Videoconferencing applications (e.g., Zoom, Microsoft Teams) can serve as functional alternatives to dedicated screen capture software for recording synchronous lectures (Stanford, 2020). Instructors can initiate private meetings to record on-screen content and audio, with or without an accompanying talking head (i.e., live video of the speaker). This approach can also extend to a wider audience and lends itself as a live, synchronous lecture option. The primary limitation of videoconferencing platforms is the lack of postcapture editing capabilities; however, their prevalence and annotation features make them a viable choice for lecture creation (Belt & Lowenthal, 2021; Grafton-Clarke et al., 2022; Kwon, 2022; Stanford, 2020).

VoiceThread, a cloud-based interactive platform, facilitates the integration of various multimedia elements (i.e., slide decks, images, audio) in the creation of video-based lectures. Instructors can accompany voiceover commentary of the uploaded content or optionally employ a talking head feature to enhance instructor presence. Moreover, this platform offers an interactive dimension for students, enabling them to contribute to asynchronous audiovisual comments to the lecture. Faculty control over their preferred level of student participation is discretionary and serviceable. As a video-based lecture application, VoiceThread helps promote a social learning environment and community building, particularly for students engaged in online nursing programs (Chen & Bogachenko, 2022; DeGrande et al., 2020; Gazza et al., 2021; Leigh, 2023; Merriam & Hobba-Glose, 2021; Smith et al., 2021; Stamps & Opton, 2019).

Presently, the most prevailing video technology used for viewing and sharing digital videos is video streaming, such as YouTube and Vimeo (Arkenback, 2023; Lewis et al., 2020). The emergence of high internet speeds has allowed for this type of video technology to become dominant and ubiquitous in how videos are viewed and distributed today (Huang et al., 2019). Video streaming refers to the continuous transmission of large, compressed video data that allows remote users to view videos over the internet asynchronously without having to download or save a video file to their computer or portable smart devices. The ability to transfer (stream) videos in this way has made video streaming an appealing and accommodating source for individuals and groups interested in disseminating video-based media and content, including the fields of education, nursing, and health care (Arkenback, 2023; Beisler et al., 2019; Huang et al., 2019).

Livestreaming, sometimes referred to as streaming, combines elements of video streaming and videoconferencing, which aims to disseminate synchronous, live content to a wider and expansive audience. The modern integration of interactive features, such as Chat, has evolved its participatory nature and community-building character to its current state. Mostly popularized by videogame users (e.g., Twitch, a platform used specifically for livestreaming), other well-established mainstream video streaming and social media platforms (e.g., YouTube, Vimeo, Twitter, Meta) and other videoconferencing software (e.g., Teams, Zoom) have recently broadened their video technological scope to support livestreaming capacities, making them viable pedagogical modalities for live, far-ranging lecture dissemination (DeGrande et al., 2020; Garcia & Yousef, 2023; Grafton-Clarke et al., 2022; Musa et al., 2021; Stephenson et al., 2023).

In recent years the emergence and proliferation of highly edited microvideos, typically under 60 seconds, popularized by TikTok and adopted by YouTube Shorts and Meta's Reels has occurred (Gapp, 2022; Garcia & Yousef, 2023). With YouTube Shorts alone garnering over 50 billion daily views, this type of video employs a massive distribution mechanism akin to traditional video streaming (Alphabet Inc., 2023). Although the utility of these short burst videos in nursing education remains unexplored today, their omnipresence and subsequent exposure to nursing students are significant and noteworthy (Gapp, 2022; Garcia & Yousef, 2023).

The development and use of video-based core didactic content progressively influenced the use of video technology in teaching psychomotor nursing skills and clinical practice (Clerkin et al., 2022; Gazza et al., 2021; Wolf, 2018). Because video technology is limited to audiovisual components and unable to offer direct hands-on experiences, learning technical skills and obtaining firsthand clinical practice can be more challenging in nursing education; however, viable and meaningful video-based pedagogical patterns focused on teaching and assessing clinical skills and other related aspects (i.e., application, clinical judgment, nurse-patient interactions) can still enhance and augment the learning experience for the remote learner (Chuang et al., 2018; Clerkin et al., 2022; Dodson, 2023; Jonassen & Yarbrough, 2021; Lee et al., 2016; Smith et al., 2022).

Expert modeling videos serve as a significant pedagogical tool for imparting clinical nursing skills, practices, and communication (Bang & Kwon, 2022; DeGrande et al., 2020; Fung, 2015; Kwon, 2022; Lee et al., 2016). The purpose of these types of videos is to showcase exemplary clinical conduct and empower students to learn through observation of real-world scenarios and witness an emulation of desired behaviors (Dinmore, 2019; Dodson, 2023; Lee et al., 2016). Another function of expert modeling videos is to expose students to patient conditions or clinical situations that may otherwise not be readily available or accessible in a real health care setting (Dodson, 2023). Varied in their focus, expert modeling videos can adopt first-person perspectives using GoPro head strap cameras or smart devices and have offered beneficial utility in medical and science labs for technical skill acquisition (Clerkin et al., 2022; Fung, 2015; Grafton-Clarke et al., 2022; Kwon, 2022; Thomson et al., 2018).

Social presence also is crucial for elevating student engagement and communication efficacy, especially in education programs primarily facilitated online. Incorporating audiovisual commentary (i.e., talking head) in online discussions or topic commentary, instructors can heighten students' learning experience and instinctively increase social presence and student willingness to engage in online or blended learning environments (Garcia & Yousef, 2023; Toulouse, 2020). Prioritizing social presence using video-based media can help establish a foundation for collaboration and teamwork and has major potential to contribute to the success and satisfaction of remote learners (Smith et al., 2021; Stanley et al., 2018; Stephenson et al., 2023).

EVIDENCED-BASED ADVANTAGES AND CHALLENGES OF THE TECHNOLOGY

Video technology has an extensive history in nursing education, and its function today offers distinct advantages and opportunities. The combination of using video-based media to innovate new teaching strategies and increased internet capacities collectively transformed the nursing education landscape and helped successfully move traditional in-person nursing programs to online platforms (Belt & Lowenthal, 2021; Gazza et al., 2021; Lockey et al., 2022; Merriam & Hobba-Glose, 2021; Smith et al., 2021; Stamps & Opton, 2019). In this context, however, video's influence on nursing education also poses challenges and disadvantages. The preponderance of nursing care addresses direct patient care, technical skills, physical presence, and hands-on clinical practice, which video cannot supply or offer (Bang & Kwon, 2022; Belt & Lowenthal, 2021; Kwon, 2022; Lockey et al., 2022; Shah et al., 2023). Despite the dichotomy of video advantages and disadvantages, the benefits of this technology outweigh the challenges in nursing.

Advantages

The most influential advantage of video-based pedagogical approaches in nursing education can be explained by Mayer's (2005) cognitive theory of multimedia learning, which posits the assertion that students learn better from (narrated) words and images together than from words alone, thus improving cognitive processing and active learning. This theoretical framework provides the underpinnings of how video is effective in nursing education (Mayer, 2017). Video-based lectures and skill demonstrations (e.g., expert modeling videos) effectually reduce cognitive load and optimize student learning by incorporating imagery (temporal contiguity), text with corresponding graphics (spatial contiguity), and emphasis on essential information (signaling) together. Video-based media can address cognitive, affective, and psychomotor learning areas that show, demonstrate, and teach nursing concepts affording students to learn better and more efficiently (Azher et al., 2023; Garcia & Yousef, 2023; Krautscheid, 2021).

The next immediate advantage of video technology in nursing education is flexibility, a transverse advantage that is shared and unanimous across video-based pedagogical modalities, video applications, and nursing programs (Barranquero-Herbosa et al., 2022; Beisler et al., 2019; Belt & Lowenthal, 2021; Dinmore, 2019; Lockey et al., 2022; Stanford, 2020; Stephenson et al., 2023). Educators benefit from a physical untethering from the classroom and the ability to curate and reuse a personal video library for future instruction (Dinmore, 2019; Krautscheid, 2021). Furthermore, video-based material from credible sources in the public domain can be readily used by instructors to augment and supplement course content. For students, flexibility is the primary advantage and reason for online and blended nursing programs sustenance, which fosters asynchronous self-direction in students' preferred environments and optimal personalized timing (Dinmore, 2019; Lee et al., 2016). Synchronous video-based lectures or sessions still offer flexibility for students by eliminating the need for physical presence while easing additional time constraints associated with commute, travel, work scheduling, or time zone differences (Grafton-Clarke et al., 2022; Huang et al., 2019). Furthermore, user controllability features, such as pause, rewind, and adjustable playback speeds, are cited as major strengths to online learning (Barranquero-Herbosa et al., 2022; Belt & Lowenthal, 2021; Dinmore, 2019; Krautscheid, 2021; Lee et al., 2016). The flexibility of closed captioning and transcription accessibility for video-based lectures also contributes and bolsters student experiences and learning outcomes while meeting Americans with Disabilities Act compliance (Beisler et al., 2019; Forbes et al., 2016). An additional merit of flexibility pertains to reportedly diminishing student anxiety levels by employing self-directed video recording for skills assessment or competency evaluation compared to the in-person performances, namely by permitting multiple attempts and the ability to refine their work (Clerkin et al., 2022; Forbes et al., 2016; Lee et al., 2016; Lewis et al., 2020; Purpora & Prion, 2018; Smith et al., 2021).

Additional major advantages of using video in nursing education relate to cost effectiveness, dissemination efficiency, and safety measures (Belt & Lowenthal, 2021; Grafton-Clarke et al., 2022). Many web-based applications and built-in video recording applications in computers and smart devices (e.g., Microsoft Stream, QuickTime, Screencastify, Twitch) are free to use or free with limited features and registered accounts, such as YouTube, and can be used in this capacity to disseminate material. Utilizing existing personal devices eliminates the need for specialized equipment and affords familiarity with function; however, considerations for more sophisticated video production equipment may be desired (Bang & Kwon, 2022; Clerkin et al., 2022; Dinmore, 2019; Lee et al., 2016). Video applications enable content delivery to a larger range of remote learners at one time and affords access to the teachings of distant specialized experts (Grafton-Clarke et al., 2022; Shah et al., 2023). As a synchronous learning opportunity, livestreaming helps conserve scarce resources and offers safety from perilous exposures and conditions (Choi et al., 2022). Segmentation of video content (i.e., the deconstruction of videos into specific learning activities) serves as a pedagogical and time management tool and offers a productive method for knowledge dissemination (Bang & Kwon, 2022; Belt & Lowenthal, 2021; Dinmore, 2019). Furthermore, future technological advancements will continue to improve storage and memory capacities to help support multiple simultaneous users and reduce the risk of damaged or lost materials (Beisler et al., 2019).

The use of video to teach tactile skills illustrates an important feature of online and blended nursing programs. Although this approach does not emulate traditional methods in nursing education, creative and thoughtful video-based pedagogical modalities can help incorporate important nursing education components for prelicensure and graduate students (Clerkin et al., 2022; Dodson, 2023; Smith et al., 2022). Video-based media enables a usable and recognizable method to keep pace with advancing modernized technologies while allowing nursing programs to achieve innovative modifications for assessment and evaluation of student clinical skills and practice (Choi et al., 2022; Dodson, 2023; Lockey et al., 2022; Smith et al., 2022; Stanley et al., 2018). Furthermore, video serves as a robust tool for evaluating clinical skills and facilitating faculty-student feedback (DeGrande et al., 2020; Lewis et al., 2020; Smith et al., 2022; Wolf, 2018). In this approach, students record exemplar techniques for competency-based assessments using personal smart devices or conventional video equipment, which are asynchronously reviewed and appraised by faculty (DeGrande et al., 2020; Forbes et al., 2016; Jonassen & Yarbrough, 2021; Lewis et al., 2020; Purpora & Prion, 2018). Faculty evaluations conducted in this way align with flipped classroom principles by encouraging individual creativity and student engagement while meeting course outcomes (Barranquero-Herbosa et al., 2022; Lockey et al., 2022). This approach fosters active learning and enables students to integrate and refine newly acquired clinical skills and expected behaviors in the advancement of clinical practice and knowledge (Belt & Lowenthal, 2021; Gazza et al., 2021; Lewis et al., 2020; Purpora & Prion, 2018).

Challenges

The role of video technology in the development of online-based nursing education programs is paramount; however, the bulk of this success resulted from immeasurable amounts of time and energy exerted by committed and dedicated faculty (Belt & Lowenthal, 2021; Gazza et al., 2021; Lockey et al., 2022; Merriam & Hobba-Glose, 2021; Smith et al., 2021; Stamps & Opton, 2019). While ongoing technological advancements emerge, the need for upgraded revisions in nursing curricular methodologies, the onus to develop and transfer knowledge, remains on faculty shoulders and presents an immensely challenging task (Dodson, 2023).

For instructors, factors such as lack of time, resources, and technical expertise are major disadvantages for instructors who want to use video technology in their course content (Arkenback, 2023; Beisler et al., 2019; Belt & Lowenthal, 2021; Dinmore, 2019). Although using contemporary video technologies is desirable and can help mitigate some time-related concerns, faculty still grapple with the overburdened complexities of selecting, integrating, and acclimating appropriate video-based pedagogical strategies with course and program outcomes (Belt & Lowenthal, 2021; Lockey et al., 2022; Smith et al., 2021). Additionally, free web-based platforms, such as YouTube, present the possibility of unintentional copyright infringement and may include unwanted advertisements or exposure to other videos that distract students or provide inaccurate information (Dinmore, 2019). Different video-based applications (e.g., VoiceThread) offer distinct pedagogical benefits, such as enhanced interactivity and multimodality; however, the time and energy required to discern these advantages can be a constraint for instructors (Chen & Bogachenko, 2022). To help allay faculty constraints, forming an interdisciplinary team of faculty, instructional designers (discovery and acclimation to new technology), information technology specialists (troubleshooting), and LMS administrators (integration) is recommended (Dinmore, 2019; Gazza et al., 2021; Krautscheid, 2021). The additional use of professional video production specialists can also be beneficial, especially if an elaborate video production is desired. Although such efforts could potentially increase costs due to the commissioning of professional editing skills and use of more sophisticated video equipment, broadening the scope of an interdisciplinary team in this way can help reduce overall time and technical skill constraints, which will allow faculty to focus more on curricular planning (i.e., script development) and student-centric content (Belt & Lowenthal, 2021; Dinmore, 2019).

For students, the key disadvantage of using video in nursing education exists primarily in online and blended nursing education programs, which involve an inherent inability to deliver direct, hands-on learning experiences (Bang & Kwon, 2022; Belt & Lowenthal, 2021; Kwon, 2022; Lockey et al., 2022; Shah et al., 2023). This challenge is universal across disciplines requiring video-based pedagogy for teaching kinesthetic skills and physical application of knowledge (e.g., natural science lab, art, music). Unless integrated with a blended or hybrid educational program, remote learners do not have the ability to practice clinical skills or hands-on techniques in person (Bang & Kwon, 2022; Kwon, 2022). Furthermore, although synchronous videoconferencing arrangements and student-directed videos are helpful in evaluating skills and practice assessments, the extra time required for students to acclimate to expectations and unfamiliar video technologies can divert student efforts away from learning objectives and potentially compromise the learning experience (Belt & Lowenthal, 2021; Jonassen & Yarbrough, 2021; Purpora & Prion, 2018).

For instructors and students, the inability to interact or communicate comparably to in-person classroom settings is challenging. In a conventional classroom where student visibility and spontaneous discussions are facilitated, synchronous videoconferencing aims to replicate such interactivity; however, the option for users to mute audio and disable video yields a significantly different experience (Belt & Lowenthal, 2021). Furthermore, in educational settings using asynchronous video-based lectures—often perceived as passive and isolating—an amplified risk of student disengagement subsists contributing to a lack of participation and interactivity (Belt & Lowenthal, 2021; Garcia & Yousef, 2023; Lockey et al., 2022). To moderate student disengagement, incorporating interactive video-based platforms (e.g., VoiceThread) can help foster more social presence and interconnection with other students and faculty (Chen & Bogachenko, 2022; Merriam & Hobba-Glose, 2021). Emerging evidence indicates that student disengagement can be combatted by pedagogical models that blend synchronous and asynchronous video elements, and the creation of more informal video-based content with a personable tone can enhance social presence and student satisfaction (Belt & Lowenthal, 2021). Increasingly now, researchers are investigating the meaningful benefits of integrating different modes of interactivity to video lectures, such as live quizzing, polling, and whiteboard annotation (Garcia & Yousef, 2023; Krautscheid, 2021; Mayer, 2017).

In nursing programs reliant on video-based program delivery, student engagement and community building can prove to be more challenging, especially when conducted asynchronously. Additional elements integrated along with video technology can help bridge these gaps by promoting interaction and social presence in an engaged learning experience for students (Chen & Bogachenko, 2022; Merriam & Hobba-Glose, 2021; Purpora & Prion, 2018; Stamps & Opton, 2019; Stanley et al., 2018).

SAMPLE CASE INTEGRATIONS

Case 1

In a hybrid baccalaureate nursing program, students enrolled in a didactic-only nursing research course received modular video-based lectures through VoiceThread embedded within an LMS. The VoiceThread lecture consisted of a PowerPoint presentation and instructor video commentary (i.e., lecture recorded displaying the instructor speaking picture in picture/talking head). Once published, interactive VoiceThread settings were applied and offered students the option to add a variety of comments asynchronously using video, audio, or text. Additionally, students were permitted to respond directly to each other's commentary, which featured a threading of comments produced by VoiceThread. Students who accessed VoiceThread lectures at different times were able to view commentary left by others and choose to continue the discussion. Moreover, the instructor also had the capacity to interact with students or offer clarification using a preferred commentary method. Table 12.2 shows how the learning objective aligned to the activity.

Case 2

In a hybrid baccalaureate nursing program, students enrolled in a fundamental nursing course are required to learn aseptic technique in an in-person lab environment prior

TABLE 12.2

Educational Map: VoiceThread Application

Objective(s)	Student Population	Implementation	Evaluation
Compare and contrast nursing qualitative and quantitative research methods	Hybrid baccalaureate nursing students	Students received a prerecorded video-based lecture on core course content using VoiceThread embedded within an LMS.	Using a predefined rubric, students were given feedback from course instructor and student peers on depth of critical analysis.

TABLE 12.3

Educational Map: Video-Assisted Skills

Objective(s)	Student Population	Implementation	Evaluation
Understand the steps in aseptic technique	Hybrid baccalaureate nursing students	Remote students observed demonstration of donning sterile gloves in a live first-person point-of-view video performance by the instructor using a head-mounted camera.	Online formative assessment comprised of multiple-choice questions in the form of a quiz.
Demonstrate competency in preparation of a sterile field	Hybrid baccalaureate nursing students	Remote students recorded a self-demonstration of sterile field preparation competency.	Using a point-based rubric, students engaged in self-assessment reports and appraised along with instructor feedback.

to advancing to more technical skills, such as endotracheal suctioning or indwelling urinary catheter insertions. For students in need of remote lab presence owing to an encumbrance, the instructor donned first-person point-of-view equipment (i.e., GoPro head-mount camera) furnished to provide livestreaming capacities using YouTube. YouTube settings were set to enforce security and privacy, then shared with remote students. In-person and remote students observed the steps of aseptic technique in first-person and third-person viewpoints simultaneously. Table 12.3 provides an example of the tool mapped to learning objectives.

Case 3

In an online graduate nursing program, adult nurse practitioner (ANP) students enrolled in an introductory advanced health assessment online course are required to learn patient interview communication skills. ANP students asynchronously viewed a video recording of an exemplar patient-centered interview performed by faculty as the interviewer and patient. The expert modeling video was used to provide context, expectations, and exhibition of therapeutic behaviors and approaches. As part of evaluating competence in interviewing communication skills, ANP students were required to submit a recording of their own mock patient interviews of consenting family members, friends, or peers. Recordings were conducted using students' preference but submitted through the institution's LMS. Table 12.4 provides an example of the tool mapped to learning objectives.

TABLE 12.4

Educational Map: Video for Communication Skills

Objective(s)	Student Population	Implementation	Evaluation
Identify key components of an effective patient-centered interview	Online advanced practice nurse (APN) graduate students	Students viewed a prerecorded expert modeling video displaying expected components and therapeutic behaviors of a patient, problem-focused interview using VoiceThread embedded in an LMS.	Rubric peer evaluations of therapeutic communication skills were described and discussed, including instructor use of VoiceThread analytics to monitor participation rates.
Demonstrate therapeutic behaviors and approaches in patient interviews	Online APN graduate students	Students recorded and submitted a mock interview of a focused patient history using personal smart devices or video capturing equipment.	Using standardized rubric, students engaged in self-assessment and peer review evaluations along with instructor feedback.

EVALUATION OF THE TECHNOLOGY

Evidence indicates that video technology is a viable and effective mode for lecture content delivery and skill demonstration evaluations (Belt & Lowenthal, 2021; Chuang et al., 2018; Huang et al., 2019; Schertzer & Waseem, 2022; Wolf, 2018). Faculty assessment of student self-directed recordings as part of achieving learning objectives (e.g., mock patient interviews, competency performances) offers faculty an efficient and successful mode for providing instructor feedback and content analysis while improving the quality of skills and training of students (Lewis et al., 2020; Schertzer & Waseem, 2022; Shah et al., 2023). Furthermore, video offers additional opportunities and insights for faculty-student discussions and objectively identifies areas of remediation. Additionally, the literature indicated a heightened level of student satisfaction associated with the utilization of video content in achieving educational objectives, especially in the context of reiteration, pacing, and accessibility (Choi et al., 2022; Lewis et al., 2020; Shah et al., 2023; Wolf, 2018).

Some aspects of video technology call for revisions or standardization because the variability in which videos are described, explained, or produced is wide ranged. Inconsistent use of talking head or picture-in-picture features and poor quality of audio or lighting of video productions have been reported to affect student learning experiences and attention span; however, addressing these concerns through relatively minor investments (e.g., external microphones) and clear communication about expectations can largely mitigate negative feedback on suboptimal video quality productions (Belt & Lowenthal, 2021; Choi et al., 2022; Dinmore, 2019; Garcia & Yousef, 2023; Lockey et al., 2022).

The mainstay reality for many video-based media productions and cloud-based applications is its dependence on high broadband speeds, and though faster internet speeds have pioneered a positive effect on video technology today, performance issues remain a common issue in online education platforms (Belt & Lowenthal, 2021). Unreliable or unstable internet connection, delayed video streaming, and interrupted audio transmission comprise the most persistent technical problems; however, minor and inconsistent technical nuisances have not been found to significantly detract from class productivity (Belt & Lowenthal, 2021). Additionally, inequitable access to faster bandwidths and other video-related resources (i.e., equipment, costs) are important considerations that need to be considered for nursing education programs that utilize web-based applications and platforms for remote learners (Belt & Lowenthal, 2021; Huang et al., 2019; Lee et al., 2016).

CONCLUSION

The integration of video technology into the contemporary landscape of nursing education has become pivotal in innovative pedagogical direction and methodology, particularly as it has helped transform and enhance online nursing curriculum delivery, clinical skill assessment, and learner engagement (Arkenback, 2023; Belt & Lowenthal, 2021; Clerkin et al., 2022; Dodson, 2023). Literature supports and affirms the efficacy of video technology in enhancing multiple learning dimensions (cognitive, affective, and psychomotor realms) in achieving nursing education outcomes (Azher et al., 2023; Garcia & Yousef, 2023; Mayer, 2017).

References

Alphabet Inc. (2023). *Alphabet A1 2023 earnings call.* https://abc.xyz/investor/static/pdf/2023_Q1_Earnings_Transcript.pdf

American Association of Colleges of Nursing. (2019). *Vision for academic nursing.* https://www.aacnnursing.org/Portals/42/News/White-Papers/Vision-Academic-Nursing.pdf

Arkenback, C. (2023). YouTube as a site for vocational learning: Instructional video types for interactive service work in retail. *Journal of Vocational Education & Training,* 1–27. https://doi.org/10.1080/13636820.2023.2180423

Azher, S., Cervantes, A., Marchionni, C., Grewal, K., Marchand, H., & Harley, J. M. (2023). Virtual simulation in nursing education: Headset virtual reality and screen-based virtual simulation offer a comparable experience. *Clinical Simulation in Nursing,* 79, 61–74. https://doi.org/10.1016/j.ecns.2023.02.009

Bang, G., & Kwon, O. Y. (2022). Real-time online point-of-view filming education for teaching clinical skills to medical students. *Korean Journal of Medical Education,* 34(3), 231–237.

Barranquero-Herbosa, M., Abajas-Bustillo, R., & Ortego-Maté, C. (2022). Effectiveness of flipped classroom in nursing education: A systematic review of systematic and integrative reviews. *International Journal of Nursing Studies,* 135, 104327–104327. https://doi.org/10.1016/j.ijnurstu.2022.104327

Beisler, A., Bucy, R., & Medaille, A. (2019). Streaming video database features: What do faculty and students really want? *Journal of Electronic Resources Librarianship,* 31(1), 14–30. https://doi.org/10.1080/1941126X.2018.1562602

Belt, E. S., & Lowenthal, P. R. (2021). Video use in online and blended courses: A qualitative synthesis. *Distance Education*, *42*(3), 410–440. https://doi.org/10.1080/01587919.2021.1954882

Chen, J., & Bogachenko, T. (2022). Online community building in distance education: The case of social presence in the Blackboard discussion board versus multimodal VoiceThread interaction. *Journal of Educational Technology & Society*, *25*(2), 62–75.

Choi, J., Thompson, C. E., Choi, J., Waddill, C. B., & Choi, S. (2022). Effectiveness of immersive virtual reality in nursing education: Systematic review. *Nurse Educator*, *47*(3), e57–e61. https://doi.org/10.1097/NNE.0000000000001117

Chuang, Y.-H., Lai, F.-C., Chang, C.-C., & Wan, H.-T. (2018). Effects of a skill demonstration video delivered by smartphone on facilitating nursing students' skill competencies and self-confidence: A randomized controlled trial study. *Nurse Education Today*, *66*, 63–68. https://doi.org/10.1016/j.nedt.2018.03.027

Clerkin, R., Patton, D., Moore, Z., Nugent, L., Avsar, P., & O'Connor, T. (2022). What is the impact of video as a teaching method on achieving psychomotor skills in nursing? A systematic review and meta-analysis. *Nurse Education Today*, *111*, 105280–105280. https://doi.org/10.1016/j.nedt.2022.105280

DeGrande, H., Acker, K., Saladiner, J., Shaver, L., & Harrel, C. (2020). Lights, camera, action! An innovative synchronous approach improving online nursing students engagement. *Nurse Educator*, *45*(5), 241–242. https://doi.org/10.1097/NNE.0000000000000759

Dinmore, S. (2019). Beyond lecture capture: Creating digital video content for online learning: a case study. *Journal of University Teaching & Learning Practice*, *16*(1), 98–108. https://doi.org/10.53761/1.16.1.7

Dodson, T. M. (2023). Use of expert modeling videos in undergraduate nursing education: A systematic review. *Journal of Nursing Education*, *62*(2), 89–96. https://doi.org/10.3928/01484834-20221213-04

Forbes, H., Oprescu, F. I., Downer, T., Phillips, N. M., McTier, L., Lord, B., Barr, N., Alla, K.,

Bright, P., Dayton, J., Simbag, V., & Visser, I. (2016). Use of videos to support teaching and learning of clinical skills in nursing education: A review. *Nurse Education Today*, *42*, 53–56. https://doi.org/10.1016/j.nedt.2016.04.010

Fung, F. M. (2015). Using first-person perspective filming techniques for a chemistry laboratory demonstration to facilitate a flipped pre-lab. *Journal of Chemical Education*, *92*(9), 1518–1521. https://doi.org/10.1021/ed5009624

Gapp, D. (2022). Using TikTok as an active learning strategy. *Nurse Educator*, *47*(5), 266. https://doi.org/10.1097/NNE.0000000000001260

Garcia, M. B., & Yousef, A. M. F. (2023). Cognitive and affective effects of teachers' annotations and talking heads on asynchronous video lectures in a web development course. *Research and Practice in Technology Enhanced Learning*, *18*, 20. https://doi.org/10.58459/rptel.2023.18020

Gazza, E. A., Theriault, L., & Oyarzun, B. (2021). Selecting media to support online learning: An interdisciplinary approach. *Computers Informatics Nursing*, *39*(2), 105–111. https://doi.org/10.1097/CIN.0000000000000664

Grafton-Clarke, C., Uraiby, H., Abraham, S., Kirtley, J., Xu, G., & McCarthy, M. (2022). Live streaming to sustain clinical learning. *The Clinical Teacher*, *19*(4), 282–288. https://doi.org/10.1111/tct.13488

Huang, R., Spector, J. M., & Yang, J. (2019). *Educational technology: A primer for the 21st century*. Springer. https://doi.org/https://doi.org/10.1007/978-981-13-6643-7

Jonassen, S., & Yarbrough, A. (2021). Integrating technology in skills lab: Using smartphones for urinary catheter validation. *Journal of Professional Nursing*, *37*(4), 702–705. https://doi.org/10.1016/j.profnurs.2021.04.005

Krautscheid, L. (2021). Untethered lecture capture: Stimulating educational affordances through technology-enhanced teaching. *Nursing Education Perspectives*, *42*(6), e176–e178. https://doi.org/10.1097/01.NEP.0000000000000771

Kwon, O. Y. (2022). Online clinical skills education using a wearable action camera for medical students. *Journal of Exercise Rehabilitation, 18*(6), 356–360. https://doi.org/10.12965/jer.2244460.230

Lee, N.-J., Chae, S.-M., Kim, H., Lee, J.-H., Min, H. J., & Park, D.-E. (2016). Mobile-based video learning outcomes in clinical nursing skill education: A randomized controlled trial. *Computers Informatics Nursing, 34*(1), 8–16. https://doi.org/10.1097/CIN.0000000000000183

Leigh, G. (2023). Using VoiceThread for clinical feedback. *Nurse Educator, 48*(2), e66. https://doi.org/10.1097/NNE.0000000000001313

Lewis, P., Hunt, L., Ramjan, L. M., Daly, M., O'Reilly, R., & Salamonson, Y. (2020). Factors contributing to undergraduate nursing students' satisfaction with a video assessment of clinical skills. *Nurse Education Today, 84*, 104244. https://doi.org/10.1016/j.nedt.2019.104244

Lockey, A., Bland, A., Stephenson, J., Bray, J., & Astin, F. (2022). Blended learning in health care education: An overview and overarching meta-analysis of systematic reviews. *Journal of Continuing Education in the Health Professions, 42*(4), 256–264. https://doi.org/10.1097/ceh.0000000000000455

Mayer, R. E. (2005). Cognitive theory of multimedia learning. In Mayer R. E. (Ed.), *The Cambridge handbook of multimedia learning* (pp. 3–48). Cambridge University Press.

Mayer, R. E. (2017). Using multimedia for e-learning. *Journal of Computer Assisted Learning, 33*(5), 403–423. https://doi.org/10.1111/jcal.12197

Merriam, D., & Hobba-Glose, J. (2021). Using VoiceThread to build a community of inquiry in blended RN-to-BSN education. *Nursing Education Perspectives, 42*(1), 44–45. https://doi.org/10.1097/01.NEP.0000000000000655

Musa, D., Gonzalez, L., Penney, H., & Daher, S. (2021). Interactive video simulation for remote healthcare learning. *Frontiers in Surgery, 8*, 713119. https://doi.org/10.3389/fsurg.2021.713119

National League for Nursing. (2015). A vision for the changing faculty role: Preparing students for the technological world of health care. Vision Series. https://www.nln.org/docs/default-source/uploadedfiles/about/nln-vision-series-position-statements/nlnvision-8.pdf?sfvrsn=1219df0d_0

Purpora, C., & Prion, S. (2018). Using student-produced video to validate head-to-toe assessment performance. *Journal of Nursing Education, 57*(3), 154–158. https://doi.org/10.3928/01484834-20180221-05

Schertzer, K., & Waseem, M. (2022). *Use of video during debriefing in medical simulation.* StatPearls Publishing.

Shah, H. P., Kafle, S., Lee, J. Y., Cardella, J., Alperovich, M., & Lee, Y. H. (2023). Livestream surgeries enhance preclinical medical students' exposure to surgical specialties. *The American Journal of Surgery, 225*(2), 432–435. https://doi.org/10.1016/j.amjsurg.2022.09.055

Smith, T. S., Jordan, J., & Li, P. (2022). Video-based interactive clinical simulation: Preparing nurse practitioner students for clinical. *Journal for Nurse Practitioners, 18*(9), 995–998. https://doi.org/10.1016/j.nurpra.2022.07.014

Smith, Y., Chen, Y.-J., & Warner-Stidham, A. (2021). Understanding online teaching effectiveness: Nursing student and faculty perspectives. *Journal of Professional Nursing, 37*(5), 785–794. https://doi.org/10.1016/j.profnurs.2021.05.009

Stamps, A., & Opton, L. L. (2019). Utilizing VoiceThread technology to foster community learning in the virtual classroom. *The Journal of Nursing Education, 58*(3), 185. https://doi.org/10.3928/01484834-20190221-12

Stanford, D. (2020). Videoconferencing alternatives: How low-bandwidth teaching will save us all. IDDblog.org. https://www.iddblog.org/voicethread-or-camtasia-when-to-use-which/

Stanley, M. J., Serratos, J., Matthew, W., Fernandez, D., & Dang, M. (2018). Integrating video simulation scenarios into online nursing instruction. *The Journal of Nursing Education, 57*(4), 245–249. https://doi.org/10.3928/01484834-20180322-11

Stephenson, C. R., Yudkowsky, R., Wittich, C. M., & Cook, D. A. (2023). Learner engagement and teaching effectiveness in livestreamed versus in-person CME. *Medical Education, 57*(4), 349–358. https://doi.org/10.1111/medu.14996

Thomson, F. C., Morrison, I., & Watson, W. A. (2018). 'Going professional': Using point-of-view filming to facilitate preparation for practice in final year medical students. *BMJ Simulation & Technology Enhanced Learning, 4*(3), 148–149. https://doi.org/10.1136/bmjstel-2017-000224

Toulouse, C. (2020). Screen capture recordings enhance connectedness among students, course content, and faculty. *The Journal of Nursing Education, 59*(9), 531–535. https://doi.org/10.3928/01484834-20200817-11

Wolf, A. B. (2018). The impact of web-based video lectures on learning in nursing education: An integrative review. *Nursing Education Perspectives, 39*(6), e16–e20. https://doi.org/10.1097/01.NEP.0000000000000389

13

Virtual Patient Simulation

Elaine D. Kauschinger, PhD, APRN, FAANP

The increasing complexity of patients' health conditions in the modern health care landscape calls for highly skilled nursing professionals. However, traditional nursing education faces barriers in consistently providing students with adequate, safe, and relevant clinical learning experiences. To bridge this gap in professional development, innovative solutions are necessary. Simulation technology offers a multitude of training aspects that real patient interactions lack, including the ability to repeat scenarios, emphasize specific diseases and clinical situations, and allow students to make mistakes in a controlled setting without risking harm to patients (Roberts et al., 2019). Virtual, mixed, and augmented reality have also been utilized as training tools across various domains (Kaplan et al., 2021). Although the field of virtual simulation in nursing education is still in its early stages, its usage is rapidly expanding (Foronda et al., 2020). The purpose of this chapter is to explore virtual patient simulation (VPS).

Simulation experiences play an important component in nursing education, providing a valuable addition to direct and indirect care in health care settings (American Association of Colleges of Nursing [AACN], 2021). According to the AACN (2021) "The Essentials: Core Competencies for Professional Nursing," clinical learning experiences can be achieved through various methodologies, including simulation and virtual technology, to enhance graduates' proficiency in their competencies. This approach aligns with competency-based education, placing students at the center of the learning experience and fostering enduring learning and behaviors.

DESCRIPTION OF THE TECHNOLOGY

Virtual simulation refers to the re-creation of reality on computer screens, where real individuals operate simulated systems and assume key roles in performing skills, making decisions, or engaging in communication (Lioce et al., 2020). Expanding on this definition, virtual reality encompasses any form of learning in an environment separate from one's present physical context (Dreifuerst et al., 2021). VPS utilizes technology to create interactive clinical scenarios that immerse students in virtual environments for simulated learning. Although VPS can take several forms, it generally includes the following components:

> ▸ Virtual characters representing patients: These virtual characters serve as the patients in the simulation.

▸ User actions: Students can engage with the virtual patient by performing various actions, such as asking health-related questions (i.e., "How long have you experienced the pain?"), conducting examinations, and observing and documenting findings.

▸ Virtual patient responses: The virtual patients respond to the user's actions, often through speech, gestures, and text, but may also exhibit other behaviors

VPS offers students a dynamic and diverse platform for real-time evaluation, diagnosis, and management (Foronda et al., 2020). To create a more realistic student experience, a progression is followed, starting with an introduction to the virtual patient and progressing through a standard clinical evaluation. For nursing students, this includes gathering patient history, conducting physical examinations, analyzing laboratory and diagnostic findings, and providing a diagnosis with a management plan. This approach facilitates an authentic and immersive learning encounter, allowing learners to transition into the role of health care professionals and apply their knowledge in practice.

EVIDENCE-BASED ADVANTAGES AND CHALLENGES
Advantages

Clinical decision-making relies on critical thinking, clinical reasoning, and clinical judgment. Virtual tools can potentially bridge the current gap in teaching clinical reasoning skills (Rothlind et al., 2021; Sim et al., 2022). Enhancing clinical reasoning skills is crucial because it involves clinicians' thought processes to formulate appropriate questions and diagnoses. It plays an important role in reducing missed opportunities for diagnosis, ultimately leading to improved patient outcomes (Plackett et al., 2021). There is evidence supporting VPS as an effective pedagogy for supporting various aspects of learning, including knowledge acquisition, skills development, critical thinking, self-confidence, and learner satisfaction (Jimenez, 2022).

VPS can be effectively utilized for training in diverse contexts, such as reducing anxiety, providing cultural training, and teaching social conversational skills, both verbal and nonverbal (Foronda et al., 2020). VPS offers nursing students a realistic and safe environment to enhance their decision-making and clinical skills (Borg Sapiano et al., 2018). In a systematic review by Kononowicz et al. (2019), VPS was found to be more effective than traditional education in improving various skills, including clinical reasoning, procedural skills, and a combination of procedural and team skills. It was also found to be at least as effective as traditional education in improving knowledge outcomes.

VPS is particularly valuable as it allows students to repeatedly practice essential but uncommon clinical scenarios (i.e., myocardial infarction) that they may not frequently encounter during their clinical training. This contributes to their proficiency in handling a wide range of situations without real-world risks. VPS offers several advantages over traditional clinical experiences and other simulation technologies. In-person simulations require significant resources, including faculty, physical space, and time, which can impede their feasibility (Brown et al., 2021). On the other hand, VPS is known for its user friendliness, adaptability, and cost effectiveness, setting it apart as a beneficial alternative to other high-fidelity simulation techniques (Brown et al., 2021).

Challenges

A recent systematic review by Shorey and Ng (2021) indicated that although virtual learning experiences are cost effective, they may lack realism. Features such as realistic patient responses and dynamic interactions are directly related to the quality of the virtual platform. For faculty and students, navigating a high-fidelity software can present challenges and cause frustration and anxiety (Nye et al., 2018). When selecting a virtual technology tool, faculty should consider the technological solutions available to them, hours of operation for technical support, and the expected response time, especially during off-hours. This is critical for students who may require additional time for assignments needing a technical support response.

The economic aspects of VPS should be considered. Implementation of VPS can involve substantial costs, including software development, hardware acquisition, maintenance, and continuous technical support. Institutions must allocate enough resources to ensure VPS program availability, functionality, and sustainability; however, compared to other high-fidelity simulation methods, VPS stands out in cost effectiveness (Brown et al., 2021).

It is important to consider diversity, equity, and inclusion issues when designing and using VPS. Without addressing these areas, VPS can limit students' learning experiences and make it difficult for them to develop the cultural competency skills necessary to care for patients from diverse backgrounds (O'Brien & Knapp, 2023). For example, students from diverse backgrounds may find that the virtual patients are predominantly of a single ethnicity, age group, or gender. Without diverse and accurate representation in VPS scenarios, students may not be prepared to interact in a culturally sensitive and competent manner with patients from different backgrounds in real-world settings. Other student access challenges may be related to students with disabilities and their ability to interact with the simulation software. Nonnative English-speaking students might face difficulties understanding or interacting with virtual patients. However, when done well, engaging with patients through VPS can increase knowledge and improve attitudes toward caring for diverse patients, including transgender patients (Altmiller et al., 2022; Altmiller et al., 2023).

SAMPLE CASE INTEGRATIONS

Faculty should be strategic in choosing VPS providers, products, and services. Selecting based purely on product demonstrations or without an examination of the comprehensive products and services required for students can result in improper VPS selection.

Numerous vendors offer VPS solutions suitable for undergraduate and graduate nursing education, including Kaplan's iHuman Patients, Elsevier's Shadow Health, and Wolters Kluwer/Laerdal's vSim for Nursing. Engaging in comprehensive discussions with the vendor is vital to ensure their products and services align with course aims and objectives and can effectively enhance the student's learning experience. Evaluating several vendors is advised to discern the pros and cons of their respective offerings.

Using iHuman VPS in a Primary Care Didactic Course

VPS using iHuman was implemented in a graduate level online primary care nurse practitioner course. Cases were chosen based on progressively developing complexity throughout the course (e.g., a patient initially presenting with stable angina would be assessed later in the course for myocardial infarction).

VPS is a pivotal tool in nursing education, enhancing learning outcomes and student engagement. To maximize its benefits, the following prebriefing process was implemented:

> **Comprehensive VPS overview:** At the course's outset, students received an in-depth introduction to VPS, setting the stage for the simulation experience.

> **Navigation skills tutorial:** Basic tutorials were provided and reviewed to ensure students are adept at navigating the VPS environment, which is crucial for a seamless learning experience.

> **Alignment with course objectives:** A discussion was provided on how the VPS cases were designed to align with course objectives, particularly in developing critical thinking abilities that would enhance their nurse practitioner (NP) skills and competencies.

> **Content information:** Students were informed that the pertinent content for each case would be included in the course content before the start of each case, so they were provided with the knowledge to be successful.

> **Safe learning environment:** Emphasizing a no-penalty approach for incorrect responses, the environment encourages exploration and learning from mistakes. Students were encouraged to revisit cases multiple times to build proficiency.

> **Scenario introduction:** Each case begins with a brief scenario introduction, setting the context and objectives for the simulation.

Debriefing process for NP students involved:

> **Synchronous Zoom sessions:** This was conducted for each case, allowing real-time communication between faculty and students. All sessions were recorded for students who could not attend live sessions.

> **Session format:** Faculty began with a brief overview of the case and objectives provided in the prebrief section. Faculty focused on challenging subject areas identified during the simulation (i.e., inclusion of pertinent subjective or objective data that most students missed). A summary of the class's overall performance was provided so students in this online environment could gauge their performance.

> **Interactive engagement:** Polling questions throughout the session were used to maintain student engagement. Students were also encouraged to post questions in the chat box, which was monitored and addressed by faculty throughout the session.

> **Timely debriefing:** Conducted within one week of the case's due date.

> **Practical application:** Discussion on how lessons from the simulation apply to clinical settings. Examples included varying medication use for the same disorder by different providers and the rationale for ordering laboratory tests to assist in the assessment of disorders.

> **Consistent debriefing agenda:** A standardized agenda used throughout the course to familiarize students with the process.

> **Ethical and clinical scenarios:** Discussion of ethical dilemmas presented in the case. Exploration of how patient assessment and management may vary in different clinical settings (e.g., primary care vs. hospital).

> **Safe environment:** Faculty stressed at each debriefing the value of students' input and the importance of self-reflection to progress in developing the NP role.

Prior to the first graded VPS, students completed a practice case in the learning mode. In the iHuman learning mode, students can delve into clinical cases and scenarios at their own speed, practicing clinical reasoning, decision-making, and critical thinking skills. Students had a maximum of three attempts to complete the case with unlimited time. First, students completed a case in learning mode with a maximum of two attempts. Then the highest grade was recorded, and students had a time limit of two hours to complete the case. A grading rubric for the case is included in Table 13.1. If students asked more than 65 questions during the history, they received a zero for that section. This was established so that students had to ask pertinent questions rather than focus on finding the answers. A SOAP note was required at the end of the case and graded as pass/fail.

For the rest of the semester, students completed the VPS cases in test mode. Test mode allows faculty to evaluate students' knowledge, skills, and interactions and assess performance and comprehension of clinical concepts. iHuman then provided individual student feedback with areas of challenge and improvement, and faculty could view overall cohort performance. Table 13.2 maps a course objective to the implementation of the technology.

TABLE 13.1

Grading Rubric for Virtual Patient Simulation Case

Section	Percentage of Total Grade
History	20
Physical exam	20
Differential diagnosis	20
Ranking of differential diagnosis	15
Laboratory tests and diagnostics	15
Science exercises	10

TABLE 13.2

Educational Map: Virtual Patient Simulation, Graduate Level

Objectives	Course Criteria	Core Curriculum Concepts	Evaluation

1. Explore the interrelationships between risk factors, screening, and lifestyle practices to enhance health promotion and disease prevention in adolescent and adult patients in primary care settings.
 	
 2. For selected health problems, analyze issues and challenges related to providing advanced practice nursing care unique to adolescent and adult patients in primary care settings.
 	
 3. Identify critical elements of evidence-based management plans for adolescent and adult patients in primary care settings that address patient and family preferences, treatment goals, and an understanding of the scope of practice of the advanced practice nurse.
	Evidence of an understanding of societal issues that impact adolescents, adults, and families
	
	 Evidence of pathophysiology, assessment, diagnostic, and management knowledge application
	
	 Evidence of incorporation of health promotion/disease prevention, family, and community concepts in virtual patient simulation cases
		Care management, contextual relevance, and professional identity formation	1. Successful completion of VPS:
			  a. Grade of at least 80%
			  b. Successful completion of SOAP note
			  c. Successful completion of history notecard
			
			 2. Active participation in online debriefing sessions

Using vSim for Nursing as Undergraduate Clinical Makeup

vSim for Nursing, codeveloped by Wolters Kluwer and Laerdal Medical in collaboration with the National League for Nursing, is a web-based VPS product. Nursing students interact with patients to collect key history and physical data and to manage the patient situation. Students can work through the scenarios at their own pace and receive a performance score. The vSim cases were updated in 2023, with greater diversity of patients and the addition of complex medical-surgical cases. The revisions also included the addition of next-generation NCLEX-style questions and SBAR (situation, background, assessment, recommendation). In 2024, a new "Clinical Judgment in Action"

TABLE 13.3

Educational Map: Virtual Patient Simulation, Undergraduate Level

Clinical Objectives	Case Objectives	Evaluation
Collect and interpret assessment and pertinent health data	Assess a patient with acute respiratory distress	Scores on vSim case by assessment and intervention student actions
Implement selected nursing interventions	Document a focused respiratory assessment	SBAR score by rubric
Evaluate patient responses to 'nursing interventions	Demonstrate appropriate management of a patient in acute respiratory distress	NCLEX item scores
	Document your nursing interventions and patient response to therapy	

enhancement introduced questions before and during the simulation; students receive immediate feedback and explanations to help them understand why the answer(s) they chose were correct or what they missed, like the exchange they would have with a good preceptor. vSim modules are available for fundamentals, medical-surgical, advanced medical-surgical/critical care, health assessment, maternity, pediatric, maternity and pediatric (combined), mental health, pharmacology, and gerontology.

vSim was integrated into an undergraduate clinical nursing course as replacement for missed clinical days, up to a maximum of two missed days in one clinical rotation. Students made an appointment with the director of simulation and scheduled a full day of in-house vSim. In advance of the scheduled simulation day, students had to complete and turn in a concept map for four patient cases that were similar to what they would see using the vSim cases.

All students were familiar with the vSim program because they had used it in their health assessment and fundamentals courses. Four medical-surgical cases were assigned, and students had a maximum time of 45 minutes to complete each case. Following the first case, students completed the SBAR activity and a series of NCLEX-style questions associated with the topic and then had to provide a verbal SBAR to the simulation director. A debrief of the case followed. The students then repeated the same process for the remaining three vSim cases. If a student did not receive a passing score on the case (as set in advance by the faculty), the student could repeat the case. As wrap-up for the clinical makeup, students had to write and submit a written SBAR note incorporating the feedback from the debrief. vSim scores from the students were incorporated into the faculty debrief to focus on areas of weakness, and the concept maps were reviewed in comparison to the vSim case to dialogue about how patients with similar symptoms but different disease processes present. Table 13.3 maps a course objective to the implementation of the technology.

EVALUATION

When evaluating a VPS platform, it is important to consider the faculty's ability to create and modify the grading rubric for each case as this promotes alignment with the course objectives and customization to cater to students' specific learning requirements. VPS allows for individual and group evaluations that faculty can incorporate as formative or summative assessment. The ability to provide objective assessment of individual features of a clinical scenario, such as physical assessment, history taking, and management, is an advantage to students' understanding of concepts and their ability to remediate. Having information about a cohort of students can also assist in evaluating gaps in the curriculum.

CONCLUSION

VPS can facilitate the development of clinical reasoning, decision-making, and critical thinking, complementing other teaching methodologies. It presents a safe, economical, and realistic learning environment, aiming to produce a workforce that caters to current patient needs. As technology progresses, we can anticipate considerable advancements in VPS marked by enriched interactivity, refined graphics, and more realistic simulations. These developments will help craft a more immersive and authentic experience, enhancing student engagement and creating a more profound sense of immersion. Incorporating artificial intelligence algorithms could lead to more dynamic and adaptable behaviors, providing a customized learning experience tailored to individual student needs.

References

Altmiller, G., Jimenez, F., Wharton, J., Wilson, C., & Wright, N. (2022). HIV and contact tracing: Impact of a virtual patient simulation. *Clinical Simulation in Nursing, 64*, 58–66. https://doi.org/10.1016/j.ecns.2021.12.005

Altmiller, G., Wilson, C., Jimenez, F. A., & Perron, T. (2023). Impact of a virtual patient simulation on nursing students' attitudes of transgender care. *Nurse Educator, 48*, 131–136. https://doi.org/10.1097/NNE.0000000000001331

American Association of Colleges of Nursing. (2021). The essentials: Core competencies for professional nursing education. https://www.AACNnursing.org/Portals/42/AcademicNursing/pdf/Essentials-2021.pdf

Borg Sapiano A., Sammut, R., & Trapani, J. (2018). The effectiveness of virtual simulation in improving student nurses' knowledge and performance during patient deterioration: A pre and post-test design. *Nurse Education Today, 62,* 128–133. https://doi.org/10.1016/j.nedt.2017

Brown, K. M., Swoboda, S. M., Gilbert, G. E., Horvath, C., & Sullivan, N. (2021). Integrating virtual simulation into nursing education: A roadmap. *Clinical Simulation in Nursing, 72*, 21–29. https://doi.org/10.1016/j.ecns.2021.08.002

Dreifuerst, K., Bradley, C. S., & Johnson, B. K. (2021). Using debriefing for meaningful learning with screen-based simulation. *Nurse Educator, 46*(4), 239–244. https://doi.org/10.1097/NNE.0000000000000930

Foronda, C., Fernandez-Burgos, M., Nadeau, C., Kelley, C., & Henry, M. (2020). Virtual simulation in nursing education: A systematic review spanning 1996 to 2018. *Simulation in Healthcare: The Journal of the Society for Simulation in Healthcare, 15*(1), 46–54. https://doi.org/10.1097/SIH.0000000000000411

Jimenez, F. A. (2022). Can virtual patient simulation be used in substitution of traditional clinical hours in undergraduate nursing education? A review of the evidence. https://evolve.elsevier.com/education/expertise/simulation-success/

virtual-patient-simulation-substitution-of-traditional-clinical-hours-undergraduate-nursing-education

Kaplan, A. D., Cruit, J., Endsley, M., Beers, S. M., Sawyer, B. D., & Hancock, P. A. (2021). The effects of virtual reality, augmented reality, and mixed reality as training enhancement methods: A meta-analysis. *Human Factors, 63*(4), 706–726. https://doi.org/10.1177/0018720820904229

Kononowicz, A. A., Woodham, L. A., Edelbring, S., Stathakarou, N., Davies, D., Saxena, N., Tudor Car, L., Carlstedt-Duke, J., Car, J., & Zary, N. (2019). Virtual patient simulations in health professions education: Systematic review and meta-analysis. *Journal of Medical Internet Research, 21*(7), e14676. https://doi.org/10.2196/14676

Lioce, L., Downing, D., Chang, T. P., Robertson, J. M., Anderson, M., Diaz, D. A., & Spain, A. E. (Eds.) and the Terminology and Concepts Working Group. (2020). *Healthcare simulation dictionary* (2nd ed). Agency for Healthcare Research and Quality. https://doi.org/10.23970/simulationv2

Nye, C., Hetzel Campbell, S., Henley Hebert, S., Short, C., & Thomas, M. (2018). Simulation in advanced practice nursing programs: A North-American survey. *Clinical Simulation in Nursing, 26*, 3–10. https://doi.org/10.1016/j.ecns.2018.09.005

O'Brien, J. M., & Knapp, G. (2023). Addressing diversity, equity, and inclusion in virtual patient simulation: A systematic review. *Nurse Education Today*, 89, 103482. https://doi.org/10.1016/j.nedt.2023.103482

Plackett, R., Kassianos, A. P., Timmis, J., Sheringham, J., Schartau, P., & Kambouri, M. (2021). Using virtual patients to explore the clinical reasoning skills of medical students: Mixed methods study. *Journal of Medical Internet Research, 23*(6), e24723. https://doi.org/10.2196/24723

Roberts, E., Kaak, V., & Rolley, J. (2019). Simulation to replace clinical hours in nursing: A meta-narrative review. *Clinical Simulation in Nursing, 37*, 5–13. https://doi.org/10.1016/j.ecns.2019.07.003

Rothlind, E., Fors, U., Salminen, H., Wandell, P., & Ekblad, S. (2021). Virtual patients reflecting the clinical reality of primary care—a useful tool to improve cultural competence. *BMC Medical Education, 21*, 270. https://doi.org/10.1186/s12909-021-02701-z

Shorey, S., & Ng, E. D. (2021). The use of virtual reality simulation among nursing students and registered nurses: A systematic review. *Nurse Education Today*, 98, 104662. https://doi.org/10.1016/j.nedt.2020.104662

Sim, J. J. M., Rusli, K. D. B., Seah, B., Levett-Jones, T., Lau, Y., & Liaw, S. Y. (2022). Virtual simulation to enhance clinical reasoning in nursing: A systematic review and meta-analysis. *Clinical Simulation in Nursing, 69*, 26–39. https://doi.org/10.1016/j.ecns.2022.05.006

14

"Escaping" from Traditional Classroom Instruction: Use of Escape Rooms in Nursing Education

Sarah E. Patel, PhD, RN, C-EFM
Emily A. Reinkemeyer, MSN, RN, CPAN
Matthew Chrisman, PhD
Christine Zimmerman, PhD, RN, CHSE

Escape rooms were created as a recreation or leisure activity that involves searching for and solving puzzles and clues within a given amount of time (Taraldsen et al., 2022). They are often team based and usually involve a specific goal, such as literally escaping from a room or solving a puzzle, and require communication, teamwork, critical thinking, and task delegation (Nicholson, 2015). There are an estimated 50,000 escape rooms worldwide, with approximately 1900 in the United States (Vianna, 2023). Most escape rooms typically follow a theme that guides their included props and puzzles. In addition to leisure time and consumer use, escape rooms are a popular educational strategy used in a variety of fields, including nursing (Reinkemeyer et al., 2022). This chapter will present a discussion of advantages and challenges with technology-based escape rooms in the classroom setting, then demonstrate cases of two escape rooms integrated into nursing education curriculum.

DESCRIPTION OF THE TECHNOLOGY

As game-based learning activities, escape rooms offer the opportunity to engage in social interaction while solving problems creatively in an active environment. Their use as a didactic learning tool in higher education has been rising in popularity over the past 10 years (Taraldsen et al., 2022). Educational use of escape rooms involves the participants achieving the game goals via educational objectives (Veldkamp et al., 2020). Participants may progress through escape rooms in a linear (solve A before solving B) or nonlinear (multiple puzzles can be solved simultaneously or in any order) fashion (Cohen et al., 2020). Structured nursing exams tend to assess individual-level skills and knowledge, and thus there is a need to incorporate education strategies such as escape rooms that involve social skills, communication, and teamwork, which are also critical to the field of nursing.

Escape rooms have successfully been integrated into nursing and other professional curricula (Reinkemeyer et al., 2022). This includes using escape rooms for clinical (e.g., medication administration, knowledge of sepsis parameters, interprofessional practice) and nonclinical (e.g., communication, teamwork, problem-solving) skills. Simulation scenarios have been especially useful in creating escape rooms in nursing. These scenarios create situations exposing students to the need to trust themselves and their teammates, work as a team, and respond to time constraints and the consequences of not working quickly enough, all of which mimic real-life health care (Taraldsen et al., 2022).

Evidence examining the use of escape rooms in nursing education is in its infancy. Two burning questions related to escape rooms in nursing education are "Do they work?" and "Are they feasible and acceptable to use?" There is evidence that among nursing and other health care–related students, including pharmacy, medicine, and occupational therapy, escape rooms can increase content-specific knowledge, skills, and attitudes and are generally found to be effective at improving educational outcomes (Reinkemeyer et al., 2022; Veldkamp et al., 2020), even more so compared to traditional classroom teaching strategies. Moreover, in terms of their feasibility and acceptability, escape rooms have been found to be enjoyable, fun, engaging, and even motivating for students. Nursing and health professional students have noted satisfaction when engaging in escape rooms as part of their education (Reinkemeyer et al., 2022). Of note, among the published literature of escape rooms in education, is the lack of criticisms reported when using this novel strategy. However, escape rooms may result in participant stress or anxiety because of time restrictions for completing tasks or puzzles or from the competition between teams trying to finish the puzzles first.

Escape room activities in education, and particularly for nursing education, have evolved beyond in-person game play by incorporating technology in a multitude of ways. Traditional escape rooms used for recreation or leisure consumer activities require participants to appear in person at a physical location. These traditional escape rooms have been modified in nursing education through the integration of high- and low-fidelity simulation scenarios. Through these simulation escape rooms, students are encouraged to integrate nursing core concepts of communication, teamwork, and critical thinking. As technology has advanced, more innovative, technology-based teaching activities have been developed, including virtual escape rooms and gamification (see Chapter 9) in higher education.

Virtual escape rooms have been developed with multiple technologies, including the use of Zoom or other online communication strategies, Google Software (i.e., Google Sites, Google Slides, Google Forms, and Google Sheets) and other online platforms, and online websites such as www.breakoutedu.com or https://virtualescaping.com/. This use of technology has enhanced immersion in the topic and narrative of virtual escape rooms (Veldkamp et al., 2020). Conducting escape rooms virtually allows for remote participants or distance learners to engage in team-based activities. Given that online nursing programs are a fast-growing option around the world, virtual escape room options enable this innovative teaching strategy to supplement more traditional nursing curricula.

EVIDENCE-BASED ADVANTAGES AND CHALLENGES OF THE TECHNOLOGY

Advantages

Escape rooms offer advantages as a teaching method in their adaptability and student engagement. Educators can utilize high-fidelity simulation technology as a physical space for escape rooms or internet technology to host escape rooms virtually. Both technologies offer advantages to educators because escape rooms can be crafted to achieve a variety of outcomes, including improved teamwork, communication, confidence, and knowledge, as well as review any content the educator desires (Reinkemeyer et al., 2022). Students find escape rooms helpful and engaging, and they report increased confidence in the targeted topics following participation in the activity (Hursman et al., 2022; Moore & Campbell, 2021).

Incorporation of an escape room with a high-fidelity simulation setting offers advantages as well. High-fidelity simulation provides the truest feel of a recreational escape room by the physical setting and puzzles or locks that can be used. Educators can focus activity on any number of outcomes, including teamwork, critical thinking, assessment, and technical skills. Options are endless using high-fidelity simulation technology, as educators can create patient cases to meet any number of learning goals. Educators can also interact with participants speaking through the simulated patient or modify the simulated patient's assessment as participants progress through the game (Sarage et al., 2021). Use of a simulation lab offers nursing educators the opportunity to watch participants complete the escape room puzzles and to use the escape room as an evaluation tool (Gutiérrez-Puertas et al., 2020).

High-fidelity simulation can incorporate an array of clinical skills, but the many puzzles and clues required to solve an escape room require all participants to communicate effectively. Therefore participants are prevented from working independent of one another, which may occur in traditional simulation experiences (Frost et al., 2020). For this reason, use of simulation settings for escape rooms can be effective at teaching nonclinical skills, including teamwork, leadership, and communication (Valdes et al., 2021). These benefits make escape rooms an excellent choice for educators creating interprofessional educational events to teach collaboration; further, the format can decrease professional hierarchies and promote collaboration (Kutzin, 2019).

Virtual adaptations of escape rooms offer many benefits for educators; these activities can be designed for synchronous or asynchronous completion, individually or in groups of any size, and are useful in engaging distance learners. Virtual escape rooms can be created with minimal cost, and once designed they can be used repeatedly with limited time commitment from educators (Hursman et al., 2022). Although tactile clinical skills cannot be incorporated into a virtual escape room, educators can utilize embedded images, audio, and videos as pieces of the game to include assessment and patient care skills within the learning outcomes. Additionally, use of breakout rooms within Zoom or other online communication platforms can allow for teamwork and communication among groups (Hursman et al., 2022). Virtual escape rooms can be conducted as a tabletop exercise in small groups, still providing the benefits of multiple groups completing the activity at the same time (Dittman et al., 2021). Tabletop, web-based, or virtually synchronous escape rooms are well suited for interprofessional education teaching collaboration and teamwork among disciplines similar to simulation-based escape rooms (Dittman et al., 2021; Fusco et al., 2023).

Challenges

Escape rooms offer a variety of benefits to participants but also come with drawbacks. The greatest disadvantage is the effort required by educators to develop the room. The structure of the game must be determined (linear, open, branching) and appropriate to the setting and participants (Eukel & Morrell, 2021). Educators must create puzzles applicable to the learning outcomes, complex enough to hold interest, and consider including distractors (puzzles or clues that do not contribute to the end goal) into the activity. Educators must also consider including possible hints if groups are unable to progress, as well as prevent opportunities to progress without completing all puzzles (such as guessing a code without solving previous puzzles). Developing all the pieces of the escape room to achieve applicable learning outcomes requires significant time. Eukel and Morrell (2021) reported approximate time commitment of 20 hours to create their classroom-based escape room (puzzles and materials).

In addition to the effort and time required for designing the escape room, the use of high-fidelity simulation requires educational training and additional time to set up, conduct, and reset the simulation lab for each group of participants (Gates & Youngberg-Campos, 2020). Time should be allotted for a prebrief to orient learners to the escape room simulation and debrief following to reinforce learning through reflection, with any additional instruction as indicated (Hawkins et al., 2020). In addition to the 20 hours dedicated to designing the escape room, Eukel and Morrell (2021) reported an additional 9 hours required to complete the setup, prebriefing, escape room simulation, debriefing, and cleanup for groups of four to five students. Furthermore, group sizes are typically limited to between three and five participants in high-fidelity simulation escape rooms because of the physical size of the simulation lab, which is often the size of a hospital room (Reinkemeyer et al., 2022).

High-fidelity simulation is a powerful educational technology but can be costly to operate and maintain. Whether educator preference or facility requirement, additional personnel may be needed to run simulation equipment. In addition to typical supplies required for simulation operation (e.g., simulated medications, procedural kids, gloves), additional supplies are needed to conduct in-person escape rooms. Typical supplies used in high-fidelity escape rooms include locks, lock boxes, created puzzles, box mazes, black lights, and notecards (Wintheiser & Becknell, 2023). These additional costs may be a significant deterrent to educators in some settings, but not a concern for others (Reinkemeyer et al., 2022).

Unlike the cost constraints related to high-fidelity simulation escape rooms, virtual-based escape rooms can be subject to technological difficulties from network outages or software errors. Users may need specific technology to access different virtual escape room platforms. Furthermore, virtual-based escape rooms can limit the engagement of users who might have visual or other disabilities. Additionally, virtual escape room tools are subject to human error, and the experience can be frustrating for students if answers are keyed incorrectly (Smith & Davis, 2021). When virtual-based escape rooms are used as a group activity, educators may struggle assessing the amount of collaboration between students (Fusco et al., 2023). Similar to high-fidelity simulation escape rooms, the development and organization of virtual escape rooms can be time intensive for educators (Davenport & Irons, 2023). However, duplication and reuse of the virtual escape rooms are minimal after the initial time dedicated to creation.

SAMPLE CASE INTEGRATIONS

Case 1: High-Fidelity Simulation Escape Room

Utilizing a high-fidelity manikin in an escape room provides a unique opportunity for students to practice skills in a competitive environment. After results from Assessment Technologies Institute (ATI) standardized testing revealed that the student population struggled with content areas related to blood transfusions, an escape room case was designed to augment that specific area for undergraduate nursing students enrolled in a medical-surgical II course. The escape room experience was included in their regular simulation day during the semester. Each group of students identified their team names and competed for the fastest time. When all students had completed the escape room, prizes were awarded for fastest time and most successful blood transfusion according to evidence-based protocol.

This particular escape room was set up to be budget friendly. It used easily obtained locks and puzzles, as well as readily available blood transfusion supplies in the high-fidelity simulation laboratory. The room was a high-fidelity room dedicated solely to the escape room. To solve this escape room, clues were presented in a linear fashion, meaning that the completion of one puzzle or clue allowed the learners to move to the next clue. It was not possible in this experience to collect multiple clues at once.

Prior to initiating the escape room experience, students were prebriefed with engagement rules and oriented to the environment. Learners were assembled in groups of four to maximize participation and to remain functional in the allocated space. Learners were given a report indicating they are to enter the lab of a famous zombie researcher who had been bitten by a zombie. After the bite, the famous researcher locked up all the equipment required to administer the cure. The students had one hour to discover and implement the cure for zombiism. Participants were allowed to ask for three hints throughout the experience. If additional hints were needed, then 5 to 10 minutes were added to the final escape time. During the report it was emphasized that "this is a truly puzzling situation, and you will need all the pieces to escape."

The first clue for the students was provided in the report. Nine puzzle pieces were hidden around the room. Completion of the puzzle revealed a drug calculation question that provided a four-digit answer. This four-digit code opened a lock on a backpack hidden in the room. The backpack contained a box of gloves, a lab values sheet for the zombie patient, and a black light flashlight. The students required all three items at different points in the experience. Subsequent clues in the room included a code revealed on the manikin with use of the blacklight (Figure 14.1), staging pressure ulcers, a cypher key matching lab values to a letter of the alphabet (Figure 14.2 and Box 14.1), an alphanumeric code on the intravenous (IV) fluid bag, a rebus puzzle giving them the password to an encrypted jump drive, and a modified letter search. As students solved each clue

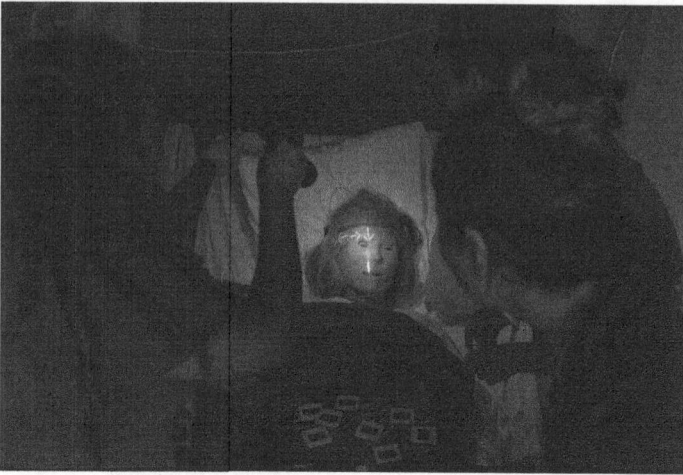

FIGURE 14.1 Blacklight Identifiable Code on the Manikin Example.

or puzzle, they identified the next puzzle and obtained essential equipment for the blood transfusion. The last two clues led them to the blood transfusion procedure and the simulated blood. Students were expected to assemble the necessary equipment and follow the procedure correctly to start the blood transfusion. Once the correct IV rate and volume were entered on the pump, the escape room had been solved.

When students successfully completed the room or one hour elapsed, the facilitator entered the room and conducted a short bedside skills debrief to ensure that all participants understood the transfusion procedure and skills. Following that, participants were relocated to the general debriefing area for a more formal simulation debrief. Discussion and reflection focused on problem-solving, teamwork, and communication. Table 14.1 includes mapping of a course objective to the high-fidelity simulation escape room.

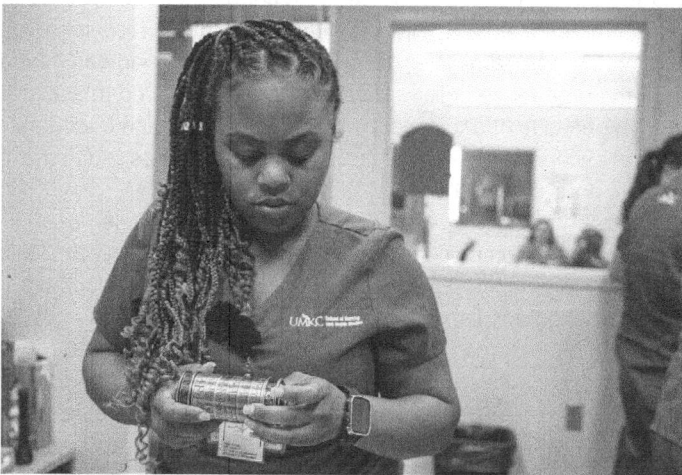

FIGURE 14.2 Cypher Lock Example.

BOX 14.1

Cypher Key by Matching Lab Values to Alphabet Example

HCT, HBG, RBC, EOS

A = 17	J =	S =
B =	K =	T =
C =	L =	U =
D =	M =	V =
E =	N =	W =
F =	O =	X =
G = .	P = 6	Y =
H = 24	Q =	Z =
I =	R =	

Evaluation of the Technology

Adding a competitive element to a traditional skill reinforcement has been very successful. Learners have reported feeling significantly more confident with blood transfusion skills and reported an increased ability to connect the content from the textbook to patient care. One of the biggest challenges in this scenario is the use of the laptop and jump drive. The current generation of learners are not exceedingly familiar with this

TABLE 14.1

Educational Map: High-Fidelity Simulation Escape Room

Objective	Student Population	Implementation	Evaluation
Identify steps to correctly initiate a blood transfusion	Prelicensure undergraduate medical-surgical II course	Small groups (max four people) will collaborate in person to solve puzzles and clues revealing supplies and procedure for blood transfusion. After successful initiation of blood, or one hour has elapsed, students will "escape."	A brief bedside review of skills occurs immediately following the end of the escape room experience regardless of success or failure in the room. Following the skills review, a structured debrief using plus/delta method and reflection occurs with a trained debriefer. Objectives related to communication, teamwork, and problem-solving are addressed at this time.

device. In the initial trial of this escape room, students paid little attention to the actual procedure and did not correctly initiate the blood transfusion. To correct this oversight, a time penalty was added for failure to follow the procedure. For each step missed or incorrectly performed, one minute was added to the final time. A warning about this was included in the procedure document. Overall, students reported a need to rely on their team members in the escape room, allowing individuals' personality and skill set strengths to shine. In addition to improved collaboration, students reported increased confidence with blood transfusing skills in the debrief. However, objective outcome data were not collected evaluating the effect of the high-fidelity simulation escape room experience on classroom performance.

Case 2: Google Form Virtual Escape Room

A maternal-newborn course integrated two virtual escape rooms utilizing Google Forms as an innovative technology medium during the COVID-19 pandemic. Prior to the pandemic, the in-person maternal-newborn course utilized paper-based case studies to facilitate learning and promote teamwork. However, these paper-based methods allowed students to preview the entire scenarios prior to applying clinical judgment skills.

Google Forms was chosen as a free online platform to create two virtual escape rooms to be used in the class: an unfolding case study as a ticket-to-class and group-based individual case scenarios based on orientation in labor and delivery triage. Students were assigned the ticket-to-class unfolding case study as a chance to asynchronously engage with the material. The first section introduced the patient scenario and trial code for students to practice "escaping." Then, students followed patient Marie's antepartum, intrapartum, postpartum, and newborn care through each room (Box 14.2). Students were allowed to use their textbook and lecture slides from the course to assist with answering the questions. By the students completing the unfolding study prior to class, students and faculty were able to identify areas requiring further clarification during class.

The second virtual escape room allowed students to work together in groups over a synchronous Zoom session. Students worked together in small groups of four to six as orienting nurses in a labor and delivery triage to review four complicated pregnancy and newborn cases. These cases included postpartum hemorrhage, preeclampsia, gestational diabetes, and jaundice in the newborn. The synchronous Zoom sessions promoted teamwork and allowed students to learn course material through discussion with peers. Table 14.2 includes mapping of a course objective to a Google Form virtual escape room activity.

Evaluation of the Technology

Focused content on healthy and complicated maternal-newborn care was presented to students in an engaging manner. Unlike a standard unfolding case study, the virtual escape room required students to successfully escape each room, which was found to be difficult even with access to course books and PowerPoints. Overall, there was a positive response from students with the integration, although students demonstrated initial frustration with case-sensitive code requirements in Google Forms. Course

BOX 14.2

Sample Escape Unfolding Case That Could Be Presented in Google Forms

Antepartum Case

Directions: After you answer each question, a number will be generated. After you have completed all the questions, enter in each of the numbers in the order of the questions. If you get each question correct, then that code will unlock the box to receive a reward.

Marie Wilson is a 32-year-old who has come to the women's health clinic after missing her period. Her last period was July 10, 2020. She reports having "frequent morning sickness" and "being unable to keep any solids down." Her blood pressure is 105/82, pulse 110, respiratory rate 22, and temperature 98.4°F. She reports pain in her lower abdomen that feels like "a sore muscle."

Question 1: Marie's pregnancy test comes back positive. Using Naegele's Rule, when is her due date?
   a. April 2, 2021
   b. March 30, 2021
   c. April 17, 2021
   d. March 16, 2021

Question 2: After confirming her pregnancy, Marie's midwife changes her chart status to G3P1011. What does G3P1011 mean?
   a. Marie has been pregnant three times with one full-term delivery and one abortion, resulting in one living child.
   b. Marie has been pregnant one time with one full-term delivery and one living child.
   c. Marie has been pregnant twice with one preterm delivery and one abortion, resulting in one living child.
   d. Marie has been pregnant twice with one full-term delivery and one preterm delivery resulting in one living child.

Question 3: Marie has returned to the clinic for her 20-week follow-up appointment. She reports a new onset of heartburn. What patient education is appropriate to give Marie? (Select all that apply.)
   a. Limit your intake of fatty foods.
   b. Eat small meals throughout the day.
   c. You may sip milk for temporary relief.
   d. Take over-the-counter calcium-based antacids that do not contain aluminum, if needed.

Question 4: At 28 weeks you are teaching Marie about kick counts. What response back from Marie indicates her understanding?
   a. I should continue kick counts for a second hour and come to the OB triage if I feel less than 10 kicks in two hours.
   b. I should count fetal movements while I walk each day.
   c. Kick counts only need to be done on a weekly basis.
   d. It is important to measure kick counts at the same time every day.

Question 5: At 32 weeks of gestation, Marie calls into the OB triage line reporting a backache with stomach tightening. What is the best nurse intervention?
   a. Take 650 mg of Tylenol.
   b. Take a warm shower to help relax your muscles.
   c. Lie down and rest for an hour.
   d. Come in to be assessed by the OB triage.

Using the code generated from your responses for each question, enter in a lock code.

TABLE 14.2			
Educational Map: Google Forms Virtual Escape Room			
Objective	Student Population	Implementation	Evaluation
Identify patient risks and complications associated with the antepartum period.	Prelicensure undergraduate maternal-newborn course	Small groups of students will collaborate on a virtual escape room over a synchronous Zoom session.	After successfully escaping the virtual scenarios or 45 minutes had elapsed, faculty and students would review the scenarios and questions. Students were provided an opportunity to ask questions for feedback on correct and incorrect answers.

faculty noted improvement in midterm examinations related to the content covered in the virtual escape rooms.

CONCLUSION

Escape rooms have become an increasingly popular educational strategy in nursing to integrate clinical and nonclinical skills (Reinkemeyer et al., 2022). The integration of high-fidelity simulation technology provides an opportunity to provide a recreational escape room feel and cost-effective solutions for varied learning needs. Although challenges exist with the implementation of escape rooms, faculty and students have reported increased confidence, communication skills, and knowledge acquisition. Escape rooms integrated in nursing curriculum provide an innovative strategy to enhance the educational environment.

References

Cohen, T. N., Griggs, A. C., Keebler, J. R., Lazzara, E. H., Doherty, S. M., Kanji, F. F., & Gewertz, B. L. (2020). Using escape rooms for conducting team research: Understanding development, considerations, and challenges. *Simulation & Gaming, 51*(4), 443–460. https://doi.org/10.1177/1046878120907943

Davenport, N., & Irons, A. M. (2024). Virtual escape rooms: Method of preparation for the next generation NCLEX. *Teaching and Learning in Nursing, 19*(1), e59–e63. https://doi.org/10.1016/j.teln.2023.08.021

Dittman, J. M., Maiden, K., Matulewicz, A. T., Beaird, G., Lockeman, K., &

Dow, A. (2021). A flexible customizable virtual escape room approach for interprofessional learners. *Journal of Interprofessional Education & Practice, 24*, 100455. https://doi.org/10.1016/j.xjep.2021.100455

Eukel, H., & Morrell, B. (2021). Ensuring educational escape-room success: The process of designing, piloting, evaluating, redesigning, and re-evaluating educational escape rooms. *Simulation & Gaming, 52*(1), 18–23. https://doi.org/10.1177/1046878120953453

Frost, K., North, F., & Smith, K. (2020). Interprofessional simulation to improve the understanding of obstetric sepsis. *Journal* for Nurses in Professional Development, 36(6), e18–e26. https://doi.org/10.1097/NND.0000000000000679

Fusco, N. M., Foltz-Ramos, K., Zhao, Y., & Ohtake, P. J. (2023). Virtual escape room paired with simulation improves health professions students' readiness to function in interprofessional teams. Currents in Pharmacy Teaching and Learning, 15(3), 311–318. https://doi.org/10.1016/j.cptl.2023.03.011

Gates, J. A., & Youngberg-Campos, M. (2020). Will you escape?: Validating practice while fostering engagement through an escape room. Journal for Nurses in Professional Development, 36(5), 271–276. https://doi.org/10.1097/NND.0000000000000653

Gutiérrez-Puertas, L., Márquez-Hernández, V. V., Román-López, P., Rodríguez-Arrastia, M. J., Ropero-Padilla, C., & Molina-Torres, G. (2020). Escape rooms as a clinical evaluation method for nursing students. Clinical Simulation in Nursing, 49, 73–80. https://doi.org/10.1016/j.ecns.2020.05.010

Hawkins, J. E., Wiles, L. L., Tremblay, B., & Thompson, B. A. (2020). Behind the scenes of an educational escape room. The American Journal of Nursing, 120(10), 50–56. https://doi.org/10.1097/01.NAJ.0000718636.68938.bb

Hursman, A., Richter, L. M., Frenzel, J., Viets Nice, J., & Monson, E. (2022). An online escape room used to support the growth of teamwork in health professions students. Journal of Interprofessional Education & Practice, 29, 100545. https://doi.org/10.1016/j.xjep.2022.100545

Kutzin, J. M. (2019). Escape the room: Innovative approaches to interprofessional education. Journal of Nursing Education, 58(8), 474–480. https://doi.org/10.3928/01484834-20190719-07

Moore, L., & Campbell, N. (2021). Effectiveness of an escape room for undergraduate interprofessional learning: A mixed methods single group pre-post evaluation. BMC Medical Education [Electronic Resource], 21(1), 220. https://doi.org/10.1186/s12909-021-02666-z

Nicholson, S. (2015). Peeking behind the locked door: A survey of escape room facilities. White Paper. https://scottnicholson.com/pubs/erfacwhite.pdf

Reinkemeyer, E. A., Chrisman, M., & Patel, S. E. (2022). Escape rooms in nursing education: An integrative review of their use, outcomes, and barriers to implementation. Nurse Education Today, 119, 105571. https://doi.org/10.1016/j.nedt.2022.105571

Sarage, D., O'Neill, B. J., & Eaton, C. M. (2021). There is no I in escape: Using an escape room simulation to enhance teamwork and medication safety behaviors in nursing students. Simulation & Gaming, 52(1), 40–53. https://doi.org/10.1177/1046878120976706

Smith, M. M., & Davis, R. G. (2021). Can you escape? The pharmacology review virtual escape room. Simulation & Gaming, 52(1), 79–87. https://doi.org/10.1177/1046878120966363

Taraldsen, L. H., Haara, F. O., Lysne, M. S., Jensen, P. R., & Jenssen, E. S. (2022). A review on use of escape rooms in education—Touching the void. Education Inquiry, 13(2), 169–184. https://doi.org/10.1080/20004508.2020.1860284

Valdes, B., Mckay, M., & Sanko, J. S. (2021). The impact of an escape room simulation to improve nursing teamwork, leadership and communication skills: A pilot project. Simulation & Gaming, 52(1), 54–61. https://doi.org/10.1177/1046878120972738

Veldkamp, A., van de Grint, L., Knippels, M.-C. P. J., & van Joolingen, W. R. (2020). Escape education: A systematic review on escape rooms in education. Educational Research Review, 31, 100364. https://doi.org/10.1016/j.edurev.2020.100364

Vianna, C. (2023). Escape room business industry statistics. https://www.xola.com/articles/escape-room-business-industry-statistics/

Wintheiser, K., & Becknell, M. (2023). A guide for facilitating an escape room for undergraduate nursing students. Teaching and Learning in Nursing, 18(1), 181–184. https://doi.org/10.1016/j.teln.2022.08.006

15

Academic Electronic Health Records

Matthew Byrne, PhD, RN, CNE

The use of electronic health records (EHRs) and other information and communication technologies have become a crucial part of health care delivery. Both prelicensure and graduate nursing students must have greater competency in utilizing these digital technologies in their care and to exercise their full scope of practice. Nursing programs and faculty have had to evaluate and integrate options for building skill and knowledge with EHRs to meet this demand. Schools of nursing and health science programs have been purchasing or creating simulated EHRs, often called academic electronic health records (aEHRs), or finding creative ways to leverage clinical EHR systems used by affiliated health care agencies. Both options expose students to a digitized patient record with health information such as past care history, allergies, medications, care plans, vital signs, assessments, care notes, and diagnostic results (e.g., laboratory values, radiology images). These systems can be utilized in the classroom, skills laboratory, and through virtual and face-to-face simulation learning experiences.

DESCRIPTION OF THE TECHNOLOGY

The aEHR market includes vendors with varying levels of functional options and a wide range of fidelity in terms of the look and feel as compared to real clinical EHR counterparts. Vendors offer a wide variety of different documentation modules, such as vital signs, care planning, and medication administration. The audience for aEHRs may include interprofessional health science students (e.g., EHR Go, MedAffinity) or may be more focused on nursing with or without linkages to vendor media such as textbooks (e.g., EHR Tutor, DocuCare, SimChart). aEHRs may be used as stand-alone teaching tools for virtual case studies and/or for simulation laboratory learning experiences with pre-, intra- and postsimulation use of the system for learning and interaction. There are also lower fidelity and functionality options available, either through vendors or even created as homegrown solutions. These lower fidelity options may be simulated documentation screens that use web-based interfaces, spreadsheets, or word processing tools that simulate portions of an EHR using options such as checkboxes and dropdowns. Some academic institutions have homegrown systems that are often built with older EHR technology or open-source systems that have varying degrees of EHR-like interfaces, functionality, and databases (e.g., Practice Fusion). No matter the fidelity and level of functionality, these systems are focused on helping students expand their clinical judgment and learn about documentation practices.

Clinical EHRs

Many students participating in clinical experiences or through telehealth may be given varying levels of access to a clinical agency's live EHR. Education programs may find that some clinical agencies will not let students access their EHRs at all versus giving them access comparable to practicing nurses (Hansbrough et al., 2020). Additionally, clinical agencies may allow on- or offsite access to training environments to allow students to learn about documentation as part of onboarding to the clinical site and in some cases for use in simulation laboratory learning experiences. Loading and resetting of training data may allow for use of affiliated agency clinical EHRs in simulation experiences or as teaching/learning tools for activities such as unfolding case studies. Several open-source EHRs have also been adopted for academic use (e.g., WorldVistA, OpenEMR, OSCAREMR).

EVIDENCE-BASED ADVANTAGES AND CHALLENGES OF THE TECHNOLOGY

The value and use of both EHRs and aEHRs as educational applications increased greatly following wider adoption of EHRs in clinical practice in the late 2000s. The Office of the National Coordinator for Health Information Technology (2023) reported that office-based adoption rates of any type of EHR was about 20 percent in 2004 compared to 88 percent in 2021. Interest and attention continued as a direct result of the COVID-19 pandemic, when many nursing and health science programs could not have students in clinical settings and needed creative ways to deliver online simulations, often with EHR as a complement. The advantages and disadvantages reflect practical issues such as costs and technical support as well as learning-based considerations such as impacts on confidence using EHRs and informatics knowledge.

The development and adoption of options for student learning related to EHRs have been examined in several studies that can help guide selection of different types of systems. Feldthouse et al. (2022) described a university and health system partnership focused on implementing a training version of a clinical EHR into simulation learning. In terms of aEHRs, Ravert et al. (2020) published a rubric for the selection of systems and an in-depth review of the selection and implementation process. Selecting and implementing systems must also be met with content and curricular integration such as use in interprofessional simulations (King et al., 2021; Schubert et al., 2022) and through strategies such as unfolding case studies (Miller et al., 2022). Surveys of aEHR users at a variety of institutions have identified the criticality of project champions and support, including program administrative support and support for students and faculty in terms of implementation and use (Badowski et al., 2018; Herbert & Connors, 2016; Raghunathan et al., 2022, 2023).

Advantages

One of the primary ways that aEHRs and EHRs are used is as a complement to simulation-based learning either through virtual simulations or in a simulation laboratory environment. Several studies support the value of EHRs/aEHRs within the context of simulation by improving decision-making and problem-solving, improved detection of safety issues, and improvement of EHR-related communications and teamwork (King et al., 2021; Nuamah et al., 2022). Evidence supporting the educational value of these systems in simulation learning experiences is critical given that all nurses will utilize EHRs in practice.

With or without simulation, both kinds of EHRs have several additional benefits for students, especially when documentation is new to them or when they are not allowed to document at clinical sites. Common benefits of using these systems included greater confidence, comfort, and skill with clinical documentation, including the digital literacy aspects of finding and interpreting data (Burrows et al., 2022; Eardley et al., 2021; Hong et al., 2022; King et al., 2021; McBride et al., 2020; Mollart et al., 2020; Raghunathan et al., 2023). In terms of digital literacy in particular, studies have validated improved critical thinking and clinical decision-making (Everett-Thomas et al., 2021; Miller et al., 2022; Mollart et al., 2020). Students also build specific clinical skills, particularly those that require an interaction between psychomotor, cognitive, and technological aspects of care, such as medication administration using bar code medication administration (Craig et al., 2021; Ledlow et al., 2022).

Using EHRs and aEHRs to learn about informatics is logical given the centrality of digital tools in health care today and the ability of these systems to model informatics concepts. Schubert et al. (2022) described an interprofessional informatics course that integrated a university's aEHR within the modules and allowed for students to see how various interprofessional roles document in the system. Kleib et al. (2021) reported a statistically significant increase in students' informatics knowledge and improvements in their documentation skills after using an aEHR, and students in that same project reported valuing practicing documentation. Repsha et al. (2020) similarly found statistically significant increases in informatics competency through use of an aEHR using the Self-Assessment of Nursing Informatics Competency Scale (SANICS) to evaluate improvement.

Challenges

Disadvantages to using aEHRs and clinical EHRs vary based on the type of system being utilized. The primary concerns noted in several recent studies are cost and faculty/student support (Badowski et al., 2018; Feldthouse et al., 2022; Herbert & Connors, 2016; Mollart et al., 2020; Raghunathan et al., 2022, 2023). The funding and cost issues stem from several aspects of selecting, implementing, and maintaining either type of system. For example, there often needs to be dedicated technical resources that can assist with the full system life cycle. System licensing costs along with dedicated support personnel can make certain options cost prohibitive. Even in cases where a teaching facility is able to use an affiliated clinical agency EHR, thus avoiding licensing costs associated with an aEHR, there can still be costs associated with loading students into the systems, learning the systems, and handling technology support issues. Many of the systems available also focus on individual learning rather than team-based or inter-professional use cases, which may limit cost sharing across health science programs or use for interprofessional education (Nuamah et al., 2022).

Support is a common issue identified in literature reviews and case studies. Extensive technical support and expertise are required through all phases of selection, implementation, curricular integration, and maintenance (Feldthouse et al., 2022; Mollart et al., 2020; Raghunathan et al., 2022). Related to this, a lack of training and support for both students and faculty (Chung & Cho, 2017; Herbert & Connors, 2016; Raghunathan et al., 2022) is a barrier given that some of these systems have technical complexities. Faculty are sometimes resistant to change (Chung & Cho, 2017; Herbert & Connors, 2016; Mollart et al., 2020) so projects may struggle if there is not ongoing faculty support or a project champion or coordinator. Even in cases where cost and faculty buy-in are not perceived as barriers, there may be a lack of faculty expertise in informatics or teaching with these kinds of systems. Expertise is required to ensure that these applications are properly integrated into the curriculum and matched appropriately to the various learning contexts in which they can be used (e.g., level of student, type of learning activities planned) (Raghunathan et al., 2022). Beyond a lack of faculty skill and knowledge, faculty also often have a lack of time and appropriate training to use an EHR/aEHR and to integrate it into the curriculum (Herbert & Connors, 2016; Mollart et al., 2020).

Students have also identified challenges such as greater time needed to extract information (Burrows et al., 2022), difficulty in using the system (Chung & Cho, 2017; King et al., 2021; Kleib et al., 2021), and a lack of familiarity with the system as compared to the clinical EHRs they have seen in practice (Eardley et al., 2021; Ledlow et al., 2022). Academic EHRs are not regulated or held to the same standards as vended, clinical EHRs. Unfortunately, this can lead to issues with content and functionality that may be outdated. For example, it has been cited that some aEHRs lack industry standard terms for gender, sexuality, and sexual orientation concepts and in some cases may contain terms that are outdated and biased (Byrne & Borzalski, 2023).

SAMPLE CASE INTEGRATION

An undergraduate baccalaureate nursing course delivered in a hybrid format required a learning module focused on care of the postsurgical patient. In the clinical case study presented, students work in a hybrid framework starting with online, asynchronous pre-work followed by a face-to-face simulation event. Students were given access to the university's aEHR to complete the first part of an unfolding case study, which includes review of a patient's record, and then begin a planned interprofessional simulation experience. During the simulation, nursing students interacted with a standardized human patient who was experiencing respiratory distress. Collaboratively, nursing and respiratory therapy students were tasked with identifying the etiology of the respiratory distress and to appropriately intervene. Students who participated in or observed the simulation were individually required to document in the aEHR flowsheets and to write a graded clinical note related to the simulation. Table 15.1 maps the technology to course objectives.

TABLE 15.1

Educational Map: Electronic Health Records

Course Objectives	Student Population	Implementation	Evaluation
Identify key patient risk factors related to postoperative complications.	Respiratory care and baccalaureate nursing students	Faculty preload a case study to be reviewed online	Prebriefing quiz the day of their simulation
Demonstrate care to a patient with emergent respiratory distress.	Respiratory care and baccalaureate nursing students	Interprofessional simulation in which a patient's respiratory state begins to deteriorate	Simulation debrief discussion on elements of interprofessional practice, communication, and teamwork
Develop a plan of care and complete documentation related to the simulation.	Respiratory care and baccalaureate nursing students	Further unfolding of patient simulation with students using the aEHR to document a plan of care and create a summary note	Rubric to evaluate the quality of student documentation using the CASE Tool (McBride et al., 2020), prioritized plan of care, and accuracy of the clinical note

As an alternative to this learning experience, students could watch a simulation event or a series of unfolding portions of a clinical case study online and then form virtual interprofessional workgroups to develop plans of care, role-based intervention strategies, and accompanying documentation.

EVALUATION OF THE TECHNOLOGY

Evaluation of EHRs and aEHRs can be viewed through different lenses. The first is evaluation of the software itself through usability evaluations and overall product evaluations, such as the rubric created by Ravert et al. (2020). Faculty and even students need to consider practical issues, such as compatibility with manikins, ability to be used by multiple students at once, or how easy it is to navigate. The second evaluation lens is how well the software improves teaching and student learning. For example, McBride et al. (2020) created the Competency Assessment in Simulation of Electronic Health Records (CASE) Tool to evaluate quality of documentation in EHR systems. Similarly, Repsha et al. (2020) used the SANICS tool to evaluate informatics knowledge after using an aEHR as a teaching tool. Researchers and faculty also used more typical assignments, such as care plans and concept maps, to evaluate if there was an improvement in students' clinical judgment and knowledge with the software serving as a mediating factor.

CONCLUSION

The use of EHRs is almost universally part of nursing clinical practice. Faculty have the opportunity to leverage aEHRs in a variety of learning contexts as a means of preparing students to work with technology in the clinical practice setting and to integrate it into their clinical decision-making process. Nursing programs considering the use of aEHRs will need to weigh factors such as cost, functionality of systems, level of administrative support, and depth of integration into the curriculum that can be achieved.

References

Badowski, D., Horsley, T. L., Rossler, K. L., Mariani, B., & Gonzalez, L. (2018). Electronic charting during simulation: A descriptive study. *Computers, Informatics, Nursing, 36*(9), 430–437. https://doi.org/10.1097/CIN.0000000000000457

Burrows, S., Halperin, L., Nemec, E., & Romney, W. (2022). Initial steps for integrating academic electronic health records into clinical curricula of physical and occupational therapy in the United States: A survey-based observational study. *Journal of Educational Evaluation for Health Professions, 19*, 24. https://doi.org/10.3352/jeehp.2022.19.24

Byrne, M., & Borzalski, C. (2023). Analysis of inclusive gender, sexuality and sexual orientation data elements in academic electronic health records. *Computers, Informatics, Nursing, 41*(12), 975–982. https://doi.org/10.1097/CIN.0000000000001064. Epub ahead of print.

Chung, J., & Cho, I. (2017). The need for academic electronic health record systems in nurse education. *Nurse Education Today, 54*, 83–88. https://doi.org/10.1016/j.nedt.2017.04.018

Craig, S. J., Kastello, J. C., Cieslowski, B. J., & Rovnyak, V. (2021). Simulation strategies to increase nursing student clinical competence in safe medication administration practices: A quasi-experimental study. *Nurse Education Today, 96*, 104605. https://doi.org/10.1016/j.nedt.2020.104605

Eardley, D., Matthews, K., & DeBlieck, C. J. (2021). Quality improvement project to enhance student confidence using an electronic health record. *Journal of Nursing Education, 60*(6), 337–341. https://doi.org/10.3928/01484834-20210520-07

Everett-Thomas, R., Joseph, L., & Trujillo, G. (2021). Using virtual simulation and electronic health records to assess student nurses' documentation and critical thinking skills. *Nurse Education Today, 99*, 104770. https://doi.org/10.1016/j.nedt.2021.104770

Feldthouse, D. M., Jacques, D. P., Fenelon, L., Robertiello, G., Pasklinsky, N., Fletcher, J., Groom, L. L., Doty, G. R., & Squires, A. P. (2022). Implementing an academic electronic health record in nursing education. *Journal of Informatics Nursing, 7*(2), 37–42.

Hansbrough, W., Dunker, K. S., Ross, J. G., & Ostendorf, M. (2020). Restrictions on nursing students' electronic health information access. *Nurse Educator, 45*(5), 243–247. https://doi.org/10.1097/NNE.0000000000000786

Herbert, V. M., & Connors, H. (2016). Integrating an academic electronic health record: Challenges and success strategies. *Computers, Informatics, Nursing, 34*(8), 345–354. https://doi.org/10.1097/CIN.0000000000000264

Hong, S., Cho, I., Park, M., Lee, J. Y., Lee, J., & Choi, M. (2022). Simulation education incorporating academic electronic medical records for undergraduate nursing students: A pilot study. *Healthcare Informatics Research, 28*(4), 376–386. https://doi.org/10.4258/hir.2022.28.4.376

King, T. S., Schubert, C., Pittman, O., Rohrig, L., McClerking, C., & Barthelmas, T. (2021). Use of an academic electronic health record with an interprofessional simulation for advanced practice nursing students. *Nursing Education Perspectives, 42*(4), 259–261. https://doi.org/10.1097/01. NEP.0000000000000621

Kleib, M., Jackman, D., Wisnesky, U. D., & Ali, S. (2021). Academic electronic health records in undergraduate nursing education: Mixed methods pilot study. *JMIR Nursing, 4*(2), e26944. https://doi. org/10.2196/26944

Ledlow, J. H., Judson, T., Watts, P., Vance, D. E., & Moss, J. (2022). Integrating a simulated electronic medical record system and barcode medication administration into a pre-licensure nursing program. *Journal of Professional Nursing, 40*, 38–41. https:// doi.org/10.1016/j.profnurs.2022.02.008

McBride, S., Thomas, L., & Decker, S. (2020). Competency assessment in simulation of electronic health records tool development. *Computers, Informatics, Nursing, 38*(5), 232–239. https://doi.org/10.1097/ CIN.0000000000000630

Miller, J., Warren, G., & Biven, S. (2022). Using the academic electronic health record to build clinical judgment skills in the classroom setting. *Teaching and Learning in Nursing, 17*(4), 438–440. https://doi. org/10.1016/j.teln.2022.05.002

Mollart, L., Newell, R., Geale, S. K., Noble, D., Norton, C., & O'Brien, A. P. (2020). Introduction of patient electronic medical records (EMR) into undergraduate nursing education: An integrated literature review. *Nurse Education Today, 94*, 104517. https://doi.org/10.1016/j.nedt.2020.104517.

Nuamah, J. K., Adapa, K., & Mazur, L. M. (2022). State of the evidence on simulation-based electronic health records training: A scoping review. *Health Informatics Journal,* 28(3), 14604582221113440. https://doi.org/ 10.1177/14604582221113439

Office of the National Coordinator for Health Information Technology. (2023). Office-based physician electronic health record adoption. Health IT Quick-Stat #50. https:// www.healthit.gov/data/quickstats/office-based-physician-electronic-health-record-adoption

Raghunathan, K., McKenna, L., & Peddle, M. (2022). Utilization of academic electronic medical records in pre-registration nurse education: A descriptive study. *Collegian, 29*(5), 645–653. https://doi.org/10.1016/j. colegn.2022.03.005

Raghunathan, K., McKenna, L., & Peddle, M. (2023). Factors in integrating academic electronic medical records in nursing curricula: A qualitative multiple case studies approach. *Nurse Education Today, 120*, 105626. https://doi.org/10.1016/j. nedt.2022.105626

Ravert, P., Whipple, K., & Hunsaker, S. (2020). Academic electronic health record implementation: Tips for success. *Clinical Simulation in Nursing, 41*, 9–13. https://doi. org/10.1016/j.ecns.2019.12.008

Repsha, C., Morse, B., Lee, S. E., Katz, J., Burrows, E., & Teates, J. (2020). Use of a simulated electronic health record to support nursing student informatics knowledge and skills. *Computers, Informatics, Nursing, 38*(2), 55–59. https://doi.org/10.1097/ CIN.0000000000000618

Schubert, C., Bruce, E., Karl, J., Nahikian-Nelms, M., Pennyman, N., Rizer, M., Vrontos, E., & Hebert, C. (2022). Implementing a novel interprofessional clinical informatics curriculum. *Computers, Informatics, Nursing, 40*(6), 411–418. https://doi. org/10.1097/CIN.0000000000000855

16

Eportfolios

Kimberly Reschke, DNP, APRN

Electronic portfolios (i.e., eportfolios) in health care education are well established likely as a direct result of the push for competency-based education (Janssens et al., 2022). A portfolio is a tool for storing, collecting, and disseminating information and supporting individuals in demonstrating knowledge, skills, and abilities in a structured way that can be easily assessed (Heeneman & Driessen, 2017; Pool et al., 2020). Eportfolios may be used for both the assessment of learning and for learning (University of Connecticut Center for Excellence in Teaching and Learning, n.d.). Within a specific class, formative assessment of portfolios can measure student performance against a course outcome, and at the end of a program a portfolio can provide evidence of program outcome achievement or summative assessment. In addition, a portfolio can be shared by the student with future employers.

DESCRIPTION OF THE TECHNOLOGY

Although paper portfolios have long been used in nursing education, advances in technology led to the development of eportfolios (Ibarra-Sáiz et al., 2020). They serve as a virtual tool for students to collect, reflect, and share learning experience and accomplishments over the course of a program, thereby aligning well to assessment of competency in a nursing program. According to a 2022 scoping review of eportfolios, competency-based education should be integrated within eportfolios to support the learning process in health care education.

There is more than one way to create or build an eportfolio. The core components should be based on the purpose and objectives for which the portfolio is designed. For example, at the simplest level, a nursing student may build a portfolio during an undergraduate program that demonstrates competency through examples of clinical rotations, preceptor and clinical evaluations, skills checklist, simulation experiences, resume, and statement of goals as a professional nurse. For a doctoral nursing student, core components of a portfolio may include (a) biographical information, (b) educational background, (c) certification(s), (d) employment history, (e) resume, (f) competency record, (g) personal and professional goals, (h) professional development, (i) presentations, consultations, and publications, (j) professional activities, (k) community activities, (l) honors and awards, and (m) letters of support (Cope & Murray, 2018).

Several learning management systems (e.g., Blackboard, Desire2Learn, Sakai, Canvas) contain portfolio tools that make it easy for students to create eportfolios. In most cases these tools incorporate web editors into templates that guide students in building their portfolios. In addition, some systems allow ways of linking assignments to an eportfolio automatically, including documents, audio files, video files, and images, among others.

In comparison, students may choose to use external platforms to create a portfolio so that it can be accessed after graduation. There are two common eportfolio platforms (Janssens et al., 2022). One platform style involves uploading and storing pieces of learning artifacts that can be easily shared with others through sites such as OneDrive, Google, or WordPress. For example, Wikispaces can be used to showcase examples of learning, and the site enables others to view, collaborate, and give feedback on the documents in a secure environment. A second platform, termed work and learn, is a more robust and interactive type, such as the tool PebblePad (Janssens et al., 2022). What makes a portfolio come alive is the ability to link to websites, videos, and other digital media. The electronic nature of portfolios makes storing and highlighting work easier but also helps to create a personal story.

The process of creating an eportfolio should be comprehensive with a clear purpose in mind. Educators need to provide guidance to their students to help them develop and utilize their portfolios effectively. To maintain a manageable and viable eportfolio process, it is important to use a simple method of completing and evaluating the eportfolio (Yancey, 2019). This can be done using rubrics, feedback, and other assessment methods and include limiting the number of criteria used to evaluate the eportfolio or creating a simple template that can be used for each portfolio (Walland & Shaw, 2022).

EVIDENCE-BASED ADVANTAGES AND CHALLENGES OF THE TECHNOLOGY

Advantages

The technology benefits of eportfolios compared to paper-based portfolios include the ease of uploading, managing, and storing examples of learning in a safe environment, often without concern for document size (Janssens et al., 2022). Students can be creative in designing their own portfolio that tells their story as a nurse, through formatting, use of electronic media, and personalization of materials. Eportfolios play a significant role in the promotion of self-awareness and self-development of students when they are encouraged to assess their own learning performance through self-reflection and facilitate the integration of theory into practice (Anderson et al., 2017). They demonstrate an individual's strengths, abilities, and experiences in nursing and show how they have grown and what they have accomplished.

Nursing students report several benefits of using eportfolios over traditional paper versions, including the ease of use and convenience, ability to get ongoing feedback, and transparency in seeing their work in the same way as others (Madden et al., 2019). Students believe the technology allows them to collect evidence in a versatile, personalized manner and creates a powerful and flexible tool to integrate both academic and practical work. Additionally, the format is more conducive to students' self-evaluation when they have more control of how material is included in the portfolio (Mollahadi et al., 2018).

Challenges

Technology can also be considered a challenge of eportfolios. Access to a safe platform to store the portfolio has been cited as a potential challenge as well as the storage capacity of the platform (Janssens et al., 2022). A recommendation to address this challenge is to evaluate eportfolio tools that have been specifically designed to meet the needs of the user. Students may not appreciate the purpose and workload related to creating an eportfolio unless that is explicitly made clear (Pool et al., 2020; Yancey, 2019).

SAMPLE CASE INTEGRATION

The use of an eportfolio in a nursing course or program should be aligned with learning outcomes. It is important to ensure that the eportfolio is used in a meaningful way and that students can reflect on their learning. It should also be used to help students develop their skills and provide feedback on their performance. Two examples are presented for consideration in Table 16.1.

EVALUATION OF THE TECHNOLOGY

When evaluating an eportfolio, multiple approaches can be taken, but evaluation is often based on the goal of the eportfolio. Defined learning objectives or competencies may support an evaluation of learning in contrast to assessment for learning where the emphasis is often centered on formative feedback and reflection. Assessment of learning is often a well-defined assignment or project over the span of a course or program, is defined by the instructor, and is summative in nature. Assessment of learning is a more

TABLE 16.1			
Educational Map: Eportfolio			
Objective(s)	Student Population	Implementation	Evaluation
Participate in ongoing activities that embrace principles of diversity, equity, inclusion, and antidiscrimination	Undergraduate baccalaureate nursing students	Students will provide a variety of evidence to support meeting this objective, such as attendance at seminars on campus, student-led events, community-based events, examples from class assignments.	Using a 10-point rubric, to what extent did the student achieve sufficient evidence to meet this objective?
Develop capacity for leadership	Graduate nursing students completing a masters or doctoral degree	Students will create an eportfolio that includes the following: personal philosophy of health, resume, examples of writing assignments, final DNP proposal, and recorded final presentation.	Rubric to assess: Melander et al. (2018)

DNP, Doctor of Nursing Practice.

student-centered approach that focuses on building a portfolio representative of that person (University of Connecticut Center for Excellence in Teaching and Learning, n.d.).

Several rubrics are available online for evaluating an eportfolio based on a set of criteria. An eportfolio rubric can be used to assess a portfolio's quality, completeness, reflection, and evidence of learning outcomes and competencies. Common features of these rubrics tend to be learner focused on criteria, such as sources of learning, demonstration of learning using artifacts, writing samples, mastery of knowledge and skills, and reflection. In an eportfolio rubric, three elements are typically included: the performance criteria (content, organization, presentation, reflection, feedback), the rating scale, and the quality indicators. The rubric in Table 16.2 is an example that can be used in the evaluation of eportfolios. It was created using several sources: EPortfolio Rubric

TABLE 16.2

Example Rubric for Electronic Portfolio-Based Assessment

Criteria	Unsatisfactory	Satisfactory	Excellent
Selection of artifacts	The artifacts do not relate to the purpose or goals of the eportfolio.	The artifacts are somewhat related to the purpose or goals of the eportfolio.	The artifacts are clearly and directly related to the purpose or goals of the eportfolio.
Reflection on artifacts	The reflections do not explain how the artifacts demonstrate learning, growth, or competencies.	The reflections explain how the artifacts demonstrate learning, growth, or competencies, but lack depth or detail.	The reflections explain how the artifacts demonstrate learning, growth, or competencies and provide evidence and examples.
Organization and navigation	The eportfolio is poorly organized and difficult to navigate. The links are broken or missing.	The eportfolio is adequately organized and easy to navigate. The links are functional and relevant.	The eportfolio is well organized and intuitive to navigate. The links are meaningful and enhance the user experience.
Design and presentation	The eportfolio is unappealing and unprofessional in its design and presentation. The layout, fonts, colors, images, and multimedia are inconsistent or inappropriate.	The eportfolio is attractive and professional in its design and presentation. The layout, fonts, colors, images, and multimedia are consistent and appropriate.	The eportfolio is impressive and creative in its design and presentation. The layout, fonts, colors, images, and multimedia are harmonious and engaging.
Writing and communication	The writing is unclear, inaccurate, or incomplete. The grammar, spelling, punctuation, and citations are incorrect or missing.	The writing is clear, accurate, and complete. The grammar, spelling, punctuation, and citations are correct and consistent.	The writing is concise, precise, and compelling. The grammar, spelling, punctuation, and citations are flawless and follow a standard style.

(Digital Portfolio Rubric), University of Wisconsin-Stout; EPortfolio Assessment Rubric, University of Tennessee at Chattanooga; Assessing ePortfolios, Educational Technologies; iRubric: A Generic Rubric for Evaluating ePortfolios and Best Practices of Using ePortfolios for Students' Learning, Reazon Systems.

CONCLUSION

Eportfolios are an effective tool for assessing learning and outcomes and for providing students with evidence of program outcomes that can be shared. Several portfolio tools are available to provide students with a comprehensive and effective way to present their learning. External platforms offer an exciting way to develop a professional portfolio that is both unique and effective. Eportfolios are an invaluable tool for both formative and summative assessments and for students to showcase their skills and knowledge.

References

Anderson, K. M., DesLauriers, P., Horvath, C. H., Slota, M., & Farley, J. N. (2017). From metacognition to practice cognition: The DNP e-portfolio to promote integrated learning. *The Journal of Nursing Education, 56*, 497–500. https://doi: 10.3928/01484834-20170712-09

Cope, V., & Murray, M. (2018). Use of professional portfolios in nursing. *Nursing Standard (Royal College of Nursing (Great Britain): 1987), 32*(30), 55–63. https://doi. org/10.7748/ns.2018.e10985

Heeneman, S., & Driessen, E. (2017). The use of a portfolio in postgraduate medical education—reflect, assess and account, one for each or all in one? *GMS Journal for Medical Education, 34*(5), doc57. https://doi: 10.3205/zma001134.

Ibarra-Sáiz, M. S., Rodríguez-Gómez, G., Boud, D., Rotsaert, T., Brown, S., Salinas Salazar, M. L., & Rodríguez Gómez, H. M. (2020). The future of assessment in higher education. *RELIEVE—Electronic Journal of Educational Research and Evaluation, 26*(1). https://doi.org/10.7203/relieve.26.1.17323

Janssens, O., Haerens, L., Valcke, M., Beeckman, D., Pype, P., & Embo, M. (2022). The role of eportfolios in supporting learning in eight healthcare disciplines: A scoping review. *Nurse Education and Practice, 63*, 103418. https://doi.org/10.1016/j.nepr.2022.103418

Madden, K., Collins, E., & Lander, P. (2019). Nursing students' perspectives on eportfolios: themes and preferences compared with paper-based experiences. *International Journal of ePorfolio, 9*(2), 87–96.

Melander, S., Hampton, D., Hardin-Pierce, M., & Ossege, J. (2018). Development of a rubric for evaluation of the DNP portfolio. *Nursing Education Perspectives, 39*(5), 312–314. https://doi.org/10.1097/01. NEP.0000000000000381

Mollahadi, M., Khademolhoseini, S. -M., Mokhtari-Nouri, J., & Khaghanizadeh, M. (2018). The portfolio as a tool for mentoring in nursing students: A scoping review. *Iranian Journal of Nursing and Midwifery Research, 23*(4), 241–247. https://doi.org/ 10.4103/ijnmr.ijnmr_195_17

Pool, A. O., Jaarsma, A. D., Driessen, E. W., & Govaerts, M. J. (2020). Student perspectives on competency-based portfolios: Does a portfolio reflect their competence development? *Perspectives on Medical Education, 9*(3), 166–172. https://doi.org/10.1007/ s40037-020-00571-7

University of Connecticut Center for Excellence in Teaching and Learning. (n.d.). *Assessing eportfolios.* https://edtech. uconn.edu/multimedia-consultation/ portfolios/assessing-eportfolios/

Walland, E., & Shaw, S. (2022). E-portfolios in teaching, learning and assessment: Tensions in theory and praxis. *Technology, Pedagogy and Education*, *31*, 2.

Yancey, K. B. (Ed.). (2019). *Eportfolio as curriculum: Models and practices for developing students' eportfolio literacy.* Stylus Publishing.

17

Working in Teams: Technology Tools for Success

Emily Chin, PhD, MSN, RNC-MNN, C-EFM

Laura Gonzalez, PhD, MSN, RNC-MNN, C-EFM

Collaboration is the essence of nursing work and, therefore, nursing education. Both virtual and in-person courses require nurses and nurse educators to employ online tools to facilitate groupwork. There are numerous choices for technology teaching aids, but adding a new or flashy gadget to an already effective teaching strategy does not always mean a better lesson. A useful starting point to weigh the utility of a tool is to consider the task, environment, and outcome desired. When considering technologies that can help students and educators collaborate, one way to approach options is to organize them by use: Is the goal for synchronous or asynchronous collaboration?

DESCRIPTION OF THE TECHNOLOGY

Synchronous Tools

Synchronous tools can facilitate a live conversation and collaboration in real time. Utilizing technology in these settings can enable audience participation or classroom engagement in both face-to-face and virtual rooms. The opportunity to provide anonymous feedback may encourage contributions. For example, Jamboard or Google Docs can allow students to answer a single question or contribute thoughts on a particular topic. Jamboard approximates a bulletin board, where individual sticky notes can be rearranged and grouped by theme. Audience response systems, such as Slido or Poll Everywhere, may also be collaborative tools. In addition to posting multiple-choice questions to query the room, audience response systems can also be used to create word clouds or lists in rank order to provide a crowd impression on a topic. In an online classroom hosted via a web-based videoconferencing platform (e.g., Zoom, Microsoft Teams), it would be easy to provide a link in the chat to quickly transport the students to the shared document or poll. In an in-person setting, sharing a link may be more cumbersome. If the links have not been provided ahead of time, directing participants to a particular page can be facilitated through providing a QR code. These can be generated through the audience response system or can be created with PowerPoint plugin software or through a third-party site, such as Bitly. In an online classroom, a main room could be divided into small groups, thus enhancing student participation and engagement. The breakout rooms are a tool to promote collaboration especially when faculty provide thought-provoking questions or activity guidelines along with time limits.

Simulations foster a safe learning environment and have proven to be adaptable, embracing collaborative technology in education. Rohrig et al. (2022) described the process for transitioning an interprofessional simulation from an in-person delivery into a virtual experience. The authors made use of prerecorded modules, Zoom conferencing, and breakout rooms to facilitate small group discussion, and they posted simulated medical records as documents to the learning management system (LMS). Standardized patients, medical equipment, and staging of medical conditions were filmed from different angles to maximize students' abilities to assess and diagnose patients. The virtual simulation offered an alternative but similar experience to an in-person interprofessional simulation. With the online platform for simulations established, there may also be growth opportunities to expand to virtual reality and technologies (Altmiller & Pepe, 2022; Rohrig et al., 2022).

Asynchronous Tools

Asynchronous tools can facilitate conversation and collaboration over a prolonged period. Tools in this category will house and organize materials that are collected over a designated period. Within each LMS (e.g., Blackboard, Canvas, Sakai) the discussion board is a natural location to begin a thread and create thoughtful dialogue around a topic or question. Individual student blogs may be a way for students to document their own thought evolution on a theme. Blogs can be hosted on the LMS or an outside site, such as WordPress. Commentary/reaction to the posts can spur discussion and collaboration. To expand beyond text-based asynchronous discussion, video sharing platforms (e.g., Panopto, VoiceThread, YouTube) allow for video elements to be an initial or ongoing conversation stimulus. Many of these tools allow for a comments section to foster reactions and a dialogue. For group projects or larger deliverables with ongoing work, office productivity software (e.g., Microsoft 365, Google Drive) can be a place where multiple students contribute to a shared document, presentation, or spreadsheet. Students may collaborate in real time, but more often they will work at their own pace, thus alleviating scheduling difficulties. For example, in preparation for each unit exam in a course, students were asked to develop one NCLEX-style question and add it to a shared Google Doc, thus creating a practice question mini-bank. After the assignment due date had passed, read-only access to the document was granted indefinitely so that students could return to the class-generated practice questions to prepare for their cumulative final. This type of collaboration lends itself equally to in-person and remote courses.

Case studies have long been an instrumental teaching tool in nursing education that has recently been adapted to include collaborative technologies (O'Mathúna, 2022; Speck et al., 2022). While teaching nursing ethics, a sometimes challenging subject to approach, technology could be used to introduce film clips, music, and art or photographs to enhance online case studies and increase engagement (O'Mathúna, 2022).

Another example of asynchronous technology tool use was with a group case study within a forensic nursing course (Speck et al., 2022). In this learning exercise, the end goal is to have a student complete an assessment and an electronic death certificate. Along the way, students interacted with an expert guest lecturer on Zoom, made several posts on the LMS discussion board, and provided peer evaluation guided by a structured rubric. Faculty responded and gave feedback through a video assessment (GoReact). This pedagogical approach was complex and creative, demonstrating a well-designed use of teaching technologies.

EVIDENCE-BASED ADVANTAGES AND CHALLENGES OF THE TECHNOLOGY

The global COVID-19 pandemic forced a rapid pivot of all nonessential activities and services, nursing education included, from in-person events to technology-enabled virtual versions (Singh et al., 2021; Speck et al., 2022). Although the volume of this transition was greatest in the pandemic years, technology use and remote collaboration have long been part of the functional reality of health care delivery and education. As with any tool, there are pros and cons to weigh when selecting a modality.

Advantages

Synchronous collaborative technology, when used well, has the advantage of bolstering engagement and facilitating conversation with quicker reactions and flowing dialogue. Collaborative technology in the form of asynchronous discussion boards, such as those hosted on an LMS, can provide time for reflection and greater freedom to share emotions and allow for quieter students to engage than might be possible in a room full of peers (O'Mathúna, 2022). Additionally, teaching with technology offers the flexibility of time and place and the ability for students to review content as desired (Singh et al., 2021; Suliman et al., 2021).

Collaborative technology used for education may begin as a way to deliver lessons, but students also develop a familiarity with the technology itself that translates into their practice careers. Many clinical sites and employers will use similar systems to deliver orientation and onboarding training. Acquainting students with their LMS, learning videoconferencing platforms, and developing skills to embrace technology are an all-around benefit to future nurses (Altmiller & Pepe, 2022).

Challenges

The advantages of educational technology use should be weighed against the challenges. Synchronous collaborative technology has a high potential for disengagement and delayed or minimal student feedback, especially if students remain muted or opt to turn cameras off (Altmiller & Pepe, 2022; Singh et al., 2021). In these cases, this lack of participation prohibits the faculty from observing the students' body language or demeanor that would be communicated in person (O'Mathúna, 2022). For both synchronous and asynchronous uses, technology accessibility may be a concern given that hardware can be costly and internet connectivity unreliable, especially in rural or underserved regions (Singh et al., 2021; Suliman et al., 2021). Additionally, health issues (e.g., eye strain, sleep disturbance, neck/back pain, headache) might result from prolonged online activity (Singh et al., 2021).

Educators surveyed by Nurse-Clarke and Joseph (2022) felt that they interacted with students less and that teaching online was less effective than an in-person version of their course. There was also a perception of a workload imbalance where online teaching required more effort; however, when administrators communicate the value of online education and back this sentiment with faculty support and opportunities for development, these concerns are addressed. Institutional support in the form of training, technological services, and resources can be leveraged to ensure that collaborative online educational tools are embraced and utilized to their maximal potential (Nurse-Clarke & Joseph, 2022; O'Mathúna, 2022; Rohrig et al., 2022).

SAMPLE CASE INTEGRATIONS

Online Synchronous Clinicals

During the height of the COVID-19 pandemic, undergraduate clinicals had to be moved from a face-to-face in-hospital setting to an online setting. Videoconferencing, such as Zoom, was used to implement virtual simulations for weekly clinicals for students. These simulations were used as an interactive group activity for the students. The instructor was able to pause the simulation and quiz the students. The students had the capacity to respond to the questions on the screen anonymously. The simulations were set up to have a different outcome depending on the options the students chose. The instructor was able to choose multiple options for each scenario to demonstrate the different outcomes if desired. Once the simulation portion of the virtual clinical was complete, the instructor and students were able to debrief and discuss what went well and what could have been done differently. Throughout the virtual simulation, the students were randomly placed into breakout rooms to work on assignments related to the clinical day. The clinical instructor was able to enter the different rooms virtually and control the time limits for the breakout rooms. The instructor was able to regroup the students in a postconference setting once they all came back from the breakout sessions. The students were then able to discuss their experience during the simulation and their group assignments. This online teaching method allowed nursing educators and institutions to continue teaching nursing students during a major pandemic in a swift and commendable way that continued to provide the necessary resources nursing students needed during the time they were not able to be in the hospital setting. Table 17.1 includes examples.

In-Person Synchronous Listening Session

During the academic year, nursing school administrators sought out bachelor of science (BSN) student council leaders to garner feedback on the program, listen to concerns, and brainstorm workable solutions. To ensure that all participants had a chance to contribute to all conversational topics and to decrease the burden on any

TABLE 17.1

Educational Map: Groupwork

Objective(s)	Student Population	Implementation	Evaluation
Sample 1 Online Synchronous Clinical			
Develop a plan of care for a virtual patient.	Undergraduate, prelicensure students in a clinical course	Virtual simulation	Debrief of the simulation experience
Sample 2 Face-to-Face Synchronous Listening Session			
Identify the most common concerns of students. Prioritize potential solutions to common concerns.	Undergraduate, prelicensure students across the BSN program	Initial discussion facilitated by question prompts Attention focused and redirected to feasible solutions by leaders in each group Comments collected and organized via shared document	Common concern themes and actionable solutions summarized by leaders and validated with student participants

one notetaker, we instituted a round-robin listening collaboration. The event was held in person, and the classroom was set up to accommodate four small groups of conversation. Each table was presented with a question prompt (e.g., clinical initiatives, diversity/equity/inclusivity, self-care, and community building) and discussion ensued for 10 to 15 minutes. At the end of this time, the question prompt cards were rotated. The question prompt card also featured a QR code, which linked to one common Google document so that notes could be taken electronically and simultaneously compiled into one location over the course of the evening. A different recorder was nominated to capture proposed ideas at each table for each round of questions. With frequent turnover and limitations of time, there was no undue burden on any one individual for the duration of the session. This round-robin approach with collaborative note-taking freed administrators and students to be present and listen to one another, allowing focus to remain on the conversation generated. This in-person team collaboration leveraged a few technological tools to maximize our time together, engage the group, and gather diverse feedback in a way that could be easily referenced and shared after the event.

This example could be replicated in several ways in the classroom, both in person and online. An unfolding case study could be presented to the class. With each scenario, small groups would each be assigned to address one portion of the nursing process, from assessment through evaluation. The collaboration means that no one person would be put on the spot and all students could benefit from working as a team. Another application of the technologically assisted round-robin discussion could be in an ethics course where students are asked to defend and debate different sides of an ethical decision. It may even be enlightening to have students take both sides of an argument and compare/contrast their evidence.

EVALUATION OF THE TECHNOLOGY

Thoughtful evaluation is necessary to determine the efficacy of teaching strategies. When using technology for collaboration, the process should match the project. For synchronous, short-term projects, a short evaluation would be appropriate. Perhaps one to two questions, either evaluating the effectiveness of the exercise or an assessment of the participant's learning, can achieve the goal. If a brief synchronous session like the example described in the previous section were replicated for the classroom, participants could be asked to scan a QR code, linking to another survey for feedback collection. For example, students could be asked to numerically rank their contribution effort to a group case study or could provide free text to describe their biggest takeaway from the discussion. With a didactic lesson, the QR code could link students to an exit NCLEX style-question evaluating the nursing knowledge gained from the session.

For longer collaborative projects using technology asynchronously, the evaluation should be more in depth. The project should begin thoughtfully with a deliberate plan to set the stage for success. Evaluation will happen through the design/development, operation, and output/disbanding stages of the project (Polyakova-Norwood et al., 2023). A well-designed project should have enough scope and variety of team roles to allow for collaborative contribution. It should also be introduced thoroughly to students so they understand the reasons for the assignment and the objectives. At the outset, a rubric (Table 17.2) should be shared with students so that they are able to understand their grading criteria. Through the operation of the collaboration, mandatory meetings with the instructor could be built in to allow for formative feedback on project progress and to allow opportunities for clarification. Checklists may be a useful tool to keep students

TABLE 17.2

Sample Grading Rubric

Criteria	3	2	1	0
Discussion participation	Student **always** has something to contribute during class time and discussion in breakout sessions.	Student **usually** has something to contribute during class time and discussion in breakout sessions.	Student **rarely** has something to contribute during class time and discussion in breakout sessions.	Student **never** has something to contribute during class time and discussion in breakout sessions.
Attitude	Student **always** has a positive attitude and is respectful toward other students' perspectives.	Student **usually** has a positive attitude and is respectful toward other students' perspectives.	Student **rarely** has a positive attitude and is respectful toward other students' perspectives.	Student **never** has a positive attitude or is respectful toward other students' perspectives.
Preparation	Student is **always** prepared for class with assignments.	Student is **usually** prepared for class with assignments.	Student is **rarely** prepared for class with assignments.	Student is **never** prepared for class with assignments.

on task and provide direction. Summative evaluation comes at the output stage of the project. The rubrics previously shared are now employed to evaluate the final project. Depending on the learning outcomes, this may be a single group grade or individual grade. Some group collaborations may also want to incorporate self and peer evaluations of contribution or offer an opportunity for groups to critique other groups' projects.

CONCLUSION

Collaboration is imperative in nursing practice and essential to nursing education, but there is no single way to achieve this. Thoughtful use of technology to facilitate collaboration can enhance the learning experience of students in face-to-face and virtual lectures and simulations. Synchronous tools (e.g., polls, Jamboard, breakout rooms) may foster live conversation and discussion between and among educators and students. Asynchronous tools (e.g., discussion boards, video platforms) can provide a supportive environment for reflection and evolution of ideas over time. Education can be transformative, especially when concepts are considered beyond the individual and incorporate community and global views. Using technology to enhance collaboration is one way an educator can make this vision a reality.

References

Altmiller, G., & Pepe, L. H. (2022). Influence of technology in supporting quality and safety in nursing education. *Nursing Clinics of North America, 57*(4), 551–562. https://doi.org/10.1016/j.cnur.2022.06.005

Nurse-Clarke, N., & Joseph, M. (2022). An exploration of technology acceptance among nursing faculty teaching online for the first time at the onset of the COVID-19 pandemic. *Journal of Professional Nursing, 41*, 8–18. https://doi.org/10.1016/j.profnurs.2022.04.002

O'Mathúna, D. P. (2022). Nursing ethics education: Thinking, feeling, and technology. *Nursing Clinics of North America, 57*(4), 613–625. https://doi.org/10.1016/j.cnur.2022.06.009

Polyakova-Norwood, V., Creed, J., Patterson, B., & Heiney, S. (2023). Making group work gratifying: Implementing and evaluating a three-stage model of group. processes in an online nursing course. *Journal of Professional Nursing, 46*, 13–18. https://doi.org/10.1016/j.profnurs.2023.02.004

Rohrig, L., Burlingame, S., Dickerson, M. B., Harter, E. A., & Justice, S. (2022). Interprofessional simulation in a digital world: Teaching collaborative practice in web-based environments. *Nursing Clinics of North America, 57*(4), 639–652. https://doi.org/10.1016/j.cnur.2022.06.011

Singh, H. K., Joshi, A., Malepati, R. N., Najeeb, S., Balakrishna, P., Pannerselvam, N. K., Singh, Y. K., & Ganne, P. (2021). A survey of e-learning methods in nursing and medical education during COVID-19 pandemic in India. *Nurse Education Today, 99*, 104796. https://doi.org/10.1016/j.nedt.2021.104796

Speck, P. M., Dowdell, E. B., & Mitchell, S. A. (2022). Innovative pedagogical approaches to teaching advanced forensic nursing. *Nursing Clinics of North America, 57*(4), 653–670. https://doi.org/10.1016/j.cnur.2022.07.004

Suliman, W. A., Abu-Moghli, F. A., Khalaf, I., Zumot, A. F., & Nabolsi, M. (2021). Experiences of nursing students under the unprecedented abrupt online learning format forced by the national curfew due to COVID-19: A qualitative research. study. *Nurse Education Today, 100*, 104829. https://doi.org/10.1016/j.nedt.2021.104829

18

The Speed of Sense Making

Matthew Byrne, PhD, RN, CNE

Rachel Onello, PhD, RN, CHSE, CNE, CNE-cl, CNL, ANEF

Michelle C. Moulton, DNP, RN, CHSE, CNE

Responding to technological innovations is not new for nurse educators who have endured waves of positive and negative technological impacts. Truly disruptive innovations, though, can accelerate the pace of technological change requiring a greater speed of sense making. Sense making is an intentional process of interpreting confusing or new circumstances by way of words, dialogue, and writing to make meaning with the purpose of taking action (Christianson & Barton, 2020). Sense making is an established concept from organizational science and behavior literature that aligns well to nursing educational models. For example, Benner et al. (2010) identified the importance of helping students with sense making, or finding a sense of saliency, within clinical scenarios to help grow their clinical judgment and decision-making. Similarly, sense-making efforts can help nurse educators find saliency with the introduction of emerging, complex, and truly disruptive innovations in teaching technology.

Ray Kurzweil (2005) famously posited that the rapidity of technological change would eventually cause "a rupture in the fabric of human history" (p. 25). Perhaps hyperbolic in the realm of educational technology, it is without exaggeration in terms of what technology has meant for humankind. In the last 50 years, human longevity has lengthened by decades largely because of medical and technological achievements. The disruptive innovations we navigate in health care can often equally impact educational and academic environments. The rapid integration of artificial intelligence (AI), process automation, and the progressive dependency on technology for nursing and educational practices are prime examples. The imperative created by these disruptive innovations in academia is to continue to prepare a clinically and technologically savvy nursing workforce that can thrive in the evolving care environment and promote quality of life in our communities.

Educators must be agile adopters and proactive analysts rather than being reactive and persistently reliant on outdated practices. Complex problems require advanced ways of knowing, thinking, and teaching and may require a rethinking of approaches to communication, collaboration, and creative problem-solving. Interprofessional dialogue has historically been a productive solution and pathway to saliency given the value of multiple perspectives and the reality that fast-moving technological innovations rarely have unilateral effects. One such approach to accelerating human and user-centered design is an input and research strategy called participatory design (PD). PD activities require end users to be directly engaged in ideation and development of new products or ideas. As the eventual end users, they are best suited to provide feedback and refine solutions to their problems. Some PD experiences can intentionally or unintentionally also enter a third space, which is a unique cognitive and communication experience in which experts and users from multiple domains enter a porous and transcendent intellectual space of cocreation. The technology encompasses "a physical, virtual, cognitive, and conceptual space where participants may negotiate, reflect, and form new knowledge and worldviews working toward creative, practical and applicable solutions, finding innovative, appropriate research methods, interpreting findings, proposing new theories, recommending next steps, and even designing solutions such as new information objects or services" (Hansen et al., 2021, p. xii).

PD and third space experiences can leverage interprofessional dialogues and expertise in new ways and can potentially help accelerate the speed of sense making required for disruptive innovations.

CASE STUDY, PART 1

The provost of Majestic Falls University has announced a summer workshop focused on generative AI. More specifically, the workshop focuses on the potential uses and challenges of generative AI applications, such as Google Bard and ChatGPT, which can produce a vast array of outputs (e.g., music, images, multiple types of written formats). The provost has asked that there be an initial gathering of pros, cons, and questions from all faculty across departments to get a sense of current thinking and concerns. Questions to consider: Which departments and stakeholders might be best for gathering this information? Are there certain groups that may offer more meaningful insights as compared to others?

Interprofessional Problem-Solving

Multiple perspectives, conceptual explorations, and experiential domains of knowledge may be needed to help break down thorny problems across academia and clinical practice. For one discipline to pursue solutions to complex problems in isolation ignores the benefit of synergistic patterns of knowing and the intertwined nature of health care delivery. New problem-solving strategies may also be required when novel technologies, such as generative AI, must be assessed and integrated within team-based, complex adaptive systems, such as health care (Pype et al., 2018). To maximize benefit and reduce harm, one approach is to engage in dynamic forms of inter- and intradisciplinary dialogues. Interprofessional education and the emphasis on well-developed interdisciplinary team communication have been focuses within health care and academia for decades (Donovan et al., 2018; Samuriwo, 2022). Improving the ways in which health care providers learn and work together has been identified as a means of addressing chronic quality and safety issues and can be equally useful to address challenges presented by technology.

In a clinical context, individual disciplines are gathered to address quality or safety issues by advocating and solutioning from their role-based perspectives. Clinicians rely on, expect, and trust each other to deliver and coordinate high-quality care within their designated scope. Maintenance of such practice and of intellectual boundaries has value in cases where role-based expectations promote safety and clarity of scope. To have blurred or overly diffuse practice boundaries may open opportunities for confusion, friction, and safety gaps. The stakes in academia may not be as high, but role integrity, differentiation, and communication are often equally important. For example, the financial aid office and an admission committee rely on each other to follow their standard practices and to maintain privacy regarding individual student situations but to openly communicate and collaborate when there are proposed changes to admission policy or procedure. Not all problems in clinical practice or academic environments, though, benefit from rigid boundaries. Beyond the basics of bringing an interdisciplinary team together, there are additional approaches to problem solving and creative ideation that may be better suited to addressing disruptive technologies. Maximal intellectual exploration and the optimal engagement by a diverse group of experts and stakeholders through PD and in some cases through third space experiences may be needed.

CASE STUDY, PART 2

The provost has asked that four workgroups assemble to address key findings from faculty feedback. The first is a faculty brainstorming and storyboarding session to examine how generative AI can be leveraged to enhance teaching, learning, and scholarship. The second is focused on administrative processes that can benefit from generative AI through promotion of efficiency and reduced administrative burden on faculty and staff. The third is a PD session focused on potential changes to the student handbook and policies related to the intersection of generative AI and plagiarism through dialogues with students, faculty, and administrators. The final workgroup will be an intentionally facilitated third space discussion with a multidisciplinary group of faculty, instructional designers, administrators, and students with a so-called blank canvas exploration of potential generative AI misuses and mitigation strategies. Questions to consider: What are the ways to best ensure productivity in these design and development formats? What individual characteristics or roles might each group consider when making recommendations of who to include?

Creating Ideas and Solutions Through Participatory Design and Third Spaces

The digitization of learning has required ongoing dialogue, reflection, and refinement of educational techniques with each progressive evolution of digital applications. When integrated and designed well, they can create greater opportunities for more holistic, accessible, inclusive, and equitable learning experiences (Araujo Dawson et al., 2022). PD is one approach to collaborative and community design in which a product or idea can be matured and evaluated to best meet the needs of users. Collective reflection, user-centered thinking, egalitarian information sharing, and the intentional engagement of diverse communities are all hallmarks of PD and reflect a power shift away from researchers/developers and toward intended end users (Bolmsten & Manuel, 2020; Hansen et al., 2021; Harrington et al., 2019). The central tenet of PD is that these end users are the most likely to be able to shape it in such a way that it best meets their needs. PD approaches include observations of product use in a laboratory or field setting, interviews and focus groups, and iterative prototyping with reflective feedback (Becker-Haimes et al., 2022; Casanova & Mitchell, 2017; Stein et al., 2016).

PD can also include a narrower scope with a guided facilitation in which end user groups enter a hybrid or third space of intersecting listening and learning (Stein et al., 2016). For situations where role boundaries and scope of practice serve as barriers to novel and progressive advancement, the traditional structure of a PD model may not be enough. When a truly novel or disruptive innovation is the goal, entering a collective space where porous boundaries and reflexive dialogue are actively cocreated can help achieve the level of disruption and novelty needed for complex problems or visionary innovations. Novel, disruptive, technological innovations may require this type of interdisciplinary third space, in which participants may be asked to let go of their roles and identities.

Third space work has been identified as an open and fertile environment for synergistic solutioning. It is often intentionally created but requires questioning of assumptions, a willingness to embrace multiple ways of knowing, and the suspension of rigid, role-defined patterns of thinking. Rather than just role-limited knowledge exchange, the focus becomes the cocreation of collective knowledge with new meaning for the purpose of sense making and transformative solutions (McAlpine & Hopwood, 2009; Sigurdardottir & Puroila, 2020).

CASE STUDY, PART 3

An external facilitator has been asked to help guide the efforts of the workgroup and to help set up a third space of collaboration for the team focused on AI misuse and mitigation strategies. The facilitator has asked for a group of individuals who demonstrate cultural awareness, openness, and skill in negotiation and democratic solutioning. The facilitator has asked for a team of eight community members with varying expertise and perspectives, including representatives from the following areas:

› English Department
› Computer Science Department
› Sociology Department
› Nursing Department
› Student Senate
› Office of Student Affairs
› Information Technology
› Instructional Design

Question to consider: What are the best ways to promote the kind of thought experimentation that reflects third spaces?

Promoting the Formation of Third Space in Participatory Design

PD and research typically occur in a workshop format in which a targeted group of stakeholders interacts with physical prototypes or ideas. The current state of a product, idea, or service is critiqued leading into an envisioning phase. The outputs (e.g., storyboards, drawings) are generated and then evaluated in the last phase for their feasibility and implementation pathways (Becker-Haimes et al., 2022; Muller & Druin, 2012). PD events in which a third space approach is desired require intentional planning, including the selection of participants with different domains of expertise; activity selection that promotes mutual learning, collaboration, and challenging of the status quo; and the logistics of time and physical or virtual spaces.

Engaging health care professionals in a role-diffuse, shared meaning-making environment may prove especially challenging. Many health care professionals have hard-fought disciplinary perspectives and entrenched advocacy stances. Asking them to step outside their intellectual comfort and practice domains may be disconcerting and difficult. The structural and power dynamics of group members, health care or otherwise, can have just as much of an impact as the individual characteristics of those participating, notably influenced by their cultural humility, cultural openness, and self-efficacy (Collins et al., 2017). The benefits of cocreation, though, parallel the benefits of true interdisciplinary practice and education; the whole of a multidisciplinary team can sometimes produce outputs greater than the sum of its individual disciplinary parts.

Although not explored in great depth within the third space literature, there are groups of professionals who may be ideal candidates. Third space professionals, notably those individuals who may work in shared academic and industry roles or whose expertise spans disciplinary and academic/industry boundaries, may bring the right characteristics to a third space session. Third space professionals, such as instructional designers and nurse informaticists, are regularly required to paradoxically hold expertise while letting go of expertise-based role boundaries to lead and translate between disciplines or industries (McIntosh & Nutt, 2022).

Hansen et al. (2021) outlined several key conditions required for third space experiences but acknowledge even with their extensive research and expertise that there is considerable room for further understanding in this area of facilitation for both PD and third space experiences. These conditions include creating physical and cognitive spaces where there is trust, guided and goal-driven shared purpose, and an atmosphere that promotes open communication and facilitates synergistic interaction. Trust is a key element of egalitarian engagement that resonates with the creation of psychological safety that is a part of nursing education, particularly when using simulation (Lackie et al., 2023). Another well-established construct used to support collaborative and diverse dialogue includes Amy Edmondson's work of psychological safety, or a "state of reduced interpersonal risk" (Edmondson & Bransby, 2023, p. 55). Participants must perceive they are in a space where they can take risks in the service of collaborating, make mistakes, share a wide range of ideas, and where their perspective is valued and heard. Psychological safety and trust can be accelerated through intentional bridging and bonding activities as well as by bringing together groups that may already have preexisting relationships or affinities.

Facilitators ultimately want to gather a group of experts who have overlapping domains of knowledge that have tensions between their roles or practice domains. A guided third space experience requires planning and outlining of the following conditions (Hansen et al., 2021):

> Intentional defining and creation of a psychologically safe space
> Definition of the problem
> Context of the problem, including the complexity and urgency
> Purpose and goals of the work
> Needs of those impacted by the problem
> Tasks, roles, and responsibilities of the group
> Facilitation of the experience
> Production of deliverables

Hansen et al. (2021) also recommended that when seeking creative codesign work in the technology space that the following groups be represented in a gathering of 8 to 10 people:

> Experts in the domain area(s) of interest who may be either stakeholders or representative of the end users or impacted audience
> Business or management representative in a codesign role
> Technical expert such as a developer or programmer in a codesign role or information source, and who may help develop the future state
> An event facilitator
> Researcher or designer that collects data

Once the format and participants are selected and trust building occurs, the real work begins. A perspective-shaping series of discussions moves from a review and critique of the current state into an effort toward revisioning the future contextualized by the problem presented. When a third space has the right participants, problem, and facilitation, there will be evidence of boundaryless dialogue, mutual learning, and cocreation of ideas for the future with full engagement from all participants. The previous content delineates the intentional work of PD and third space experiences, but there is also value in considering that third spaces can also form organically and through a self-organization process often centered on a common goal, need, or problem.

CASE STUDY, PART 4

The facilitator gathered the participants at an off-campus meeting site. The group was eager to discuss their experiences with generative AI and how it might shape student learning and the dynamics of the student-faculty relationship. Several members of the group had been part of a technology strategic committee so their preexisting relationship set a positive and collaborative tone. The facilitator posed a series of questions that resulted in a wide-ranging dialogue in which all attendees shared insights and began to formulate a new student and faculty framework related to emerging technologies and how they should be addressed as a part of the mutual learning experience. The group formulated statements that would become part of a mutual technology conduct pledge that students and faculty would discuss and sign at the start of all courses. Questions to consider: How will the third space outputs be operationalized? What additional dialogues may be needed for areas that require further exploration?

CONCLUSION

There is little doubt that technology has and will continue to have unpredictable and unprecedented impacts on health care and nursing education. Not every application or technology enhancement will fall into the category of a disruptive innovation, but they all should be evaluated for their level of impact at the intra- and interdisciplinary levels. Disruptive innovations are particularly complex by nature and may require equally innovative solutioning approaches that may benefit from multidisciplinary dialogue and expertise. Nurse educators must accelerate their speed of sense making when it comes to understanding the utility, risks, and benefits of new and emerging educational technologies. Whether the impacts are large, small, positive, or negative, adaptation is inevitable and may require new approaches, such as PD and the facilitation of third space information, to ensure proactive responses. These approaches promote a more dynamic, user-centered, inclusive, and collaborative option that can yield faster and more innovative responses and promote empowerment for all stakeholders, notably nurse educators and students.

References

Araujo Dawson, B., Kilgore, W., & Rawcliffe, R. (2022). Strategies for creating inclusive learning environments through a social justice lens. *Journal of Educational Research and Practice, 12*. https://doi.org/10.5590/JERAP.2022.12.0.02

Becker-Haimes, E. M., Ramesh, B., Buck, J. E., Nuske, H. J., Zentgraf, K. A., Stewart, R. E., Buttenheim, A., & Mandell, D. S. (2022). Comparing output from two methods of participatory design for developing implementation strategies: Traditional contextual inquiry vs. rapid crowd sourcing. *Implementation Science, 17*(1), 46. https://doi.org/10.1186/s13012-022-01220-9

Benner, P., Sutphen, M., Leonard, V., & Day, L. (2010). *Educating nurses: A call for radical transformation.* Jossey-Bass.

Bolmsten, J., & Manuel, M. E. (2020). Sustainable participatory processes of education technology development. *Educational Technology Research & Development,* 68(5), 2705–2728. https://doi.org/10.1007/s11423-020-09803-3

Casanova, D., & Mitchell, P. (2017). The cube and the poppy flower: Participatory approaches for designing technology-enhanced learning spaces. *Journal of Learning Spaces, 6*(3), 1–12.

Christianson, M. K., & Barton, M. A. (2020). Sensemaking in the time of cOVID-19. *Journal of Management Studies, 58*(2), 572–576. https://doi.org/10.1111/joms.12658

Collins, N., Chou, Y. M., Warner, M., & Rowley, C. (2017). Human factors in East Asian virtual teamwork: A comparative study of Indonesia, Taiwan and Vietnam. *International Journal of Human Resource Management, 28*(10), 1475–1498. https://doi.org/10.1080/09585192.2015.1089064

Donovan AL, Aldrich JM, Gross AK, Barchas DM, Thornton KC, Schell-Chaple HM,

Gropper MA, Lipshutz AKM; University of California, San Francisco Critical Care Innovations Group. Interprofessional Care and Teamwork in the ICU. *Crit Care Med.* 2018 Jun;46(6):980-990. https://doi.org/10.1097/CCM.0000000000003067. PMID: 29521716.

Edmondson, A. C., & Bransby, D. P. (2023). Psychological safety comes of age: Observed themes in an established literature. *Annual Review of Organizational Psychology and Organizational Behavior, 10*, 55–78. https://doi.org/10.1146/annurev-orgpsych-120920-055217

Hansen, P., Fourie, I., & Meyer, A. (2021). *Third space, information sharing, and participatory design.* Springer International Publishing.

Harrington, C., Erete, S., & Piper, A. M. (2019). Deconstructing community-based collaborative design: Towards more equitable participatory design engagements. *Proceedings of the ACM on Human-Computer Interaction, 3*(CSCW; art. no. 216), 1–25. https://doi.org/10.1145/3359318

Kurzweil, R. (2005). *The singularity is near: When humans transcend biology.* Viking.

Lackie, K., Hayward, K., Ayn, C., Stilwell, P., Lane, J., Andrews, C., Dutton, T., Ferkol, D., Harris, J., Houk, S., Pendergast, N., Persaud, D., Thillaye, J., Mills, J., Grant, S., & Munroe, A. (2023). Creating psychological safety in interprofessional simulation for health professional learners: A scoping review of the barriers and enablers. *Journal of Interprofessional Care, 37*(2), 187–202. https://doi.org/10.1080/13561820.2022.2052269

McAlpine, L., & Hopwood, N. (2009). 'Third spaces': A useful developmental lens? *International Journal for Academic Development,* 14(2), 159–162. https://doi.org/10.1080/13601440902970072

McIntosh, E., & Nutt, D. (Eds.). (2022). The Impact of the Integrated Practitioner in Higher Education: Studies in Third Space Professionalism (1st ed.). Routledge. https://doi.org/10.4324/9781003037569

Muller, M., & Druin, A. (2012). Participatory design: The third space in HCI. In Jacko J. (Ed.), *The human–computer interaction handbook* (3rd ed., pp. 1125–1154). Lawrence Erlbaum.

Pype, P., Mertens, F., Helewaut, F., & Krystallidou, D. (2018). Healthcare teams as complex adaptive systems: Understanding team behavior through team members' perception of interpersonal interaction. *BMC Health Services Research, 18*(1), 570. https://doi.org/10.1186/s12913-018-3392-3

Samuriwo, R. (2022). Interprofessional collaboration—Time for a new theory of action? *Frontiers in Medicine, 9*, 876715. https://doi.org/10.3389/fmed.2022.876715

Sigurdardottir, I., & Puroila, A.-M. (2020). Encounters in the third space: Constructing the researcher's role in collaborative action research. *Educational Action Research, 28*(1), 83–97. https://doi.org/10.1080/09650792.2018.1507832

Stein, M., Boden, A., Hornung, D., & Wulf, V. (2016). Third spaces in the age of IoT: A study on participatory design of complex systems. In M. Garschall, T. Hamm, D. Hornung, C. Müller, K. Neureiter, M. Schorch, & L. van Velsen (Eds.), *International reports on socio-informatics (IRSI), Proceedings of the COOP 2016 symposium on challenges and experiences in designing for an ageing society. Reflecting on concepts of age(ing) and communication practices.* https://api.semanticscholar.org/CorpusID:221209628